Intimate
Wars

Intimate
Wars

**The Life and Times of the Woman
Who Brought Abortion from
the Back Alley to the Board Room**

Merle
Hoffman

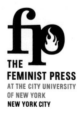

**THE
FEMINIST PRESS**
AT THE CITY UNIVERSITY
OF NEW YORK
NEW YORK CITY

Published in 2012 by the Feminist Press
at the City University of New York
The Graduate Center
365 Fifth Avenue, Suite 5406
New York, NY 10016

feministpress.org

First printing January 2012

Cover design by Herb Thornby, herbthornby.com
Text design by Drew Stevens

Library of Congress Cataloging-in-Publication Data

Hoffman, Merle, 1946–
  Intimate wars : the life and times of the woman who brought abortion from
the back alley to the board room / Merle Hoffman.
    p. ; cm.
  Includes bibliographical references and index.
  ISBN 978-1-55861-751-3 (pbk.)
  1. Pro-choice movement—United States. 2. Women's rights—United States.
3. Hoffman, Merle, 1946– 4. Feminism—United States. I. Title.
  [DNLM: 1. Hoffman, Merle, 1946– 2. Abortion, Legal--United States—
Autobiography. 3. Women's Rights--United States--Autobiography.
4. Abortion, Legal—history—United States. 5. Feminism—United States—
Autobiography. 6. Feminism—history—United States. 7. History, 20th
Century—United States. 8. History, 21st Century—United States.
9. Women's Rights—history—United States. WZ 100]
  HQ767.5.U5H64 2012
  363.46092—dc23
  [B]

                                                          2011014832

In loving memory of
Ruth Dubow Hoffman,
Jack Hoffman,
Martin Gold,
Mahin Hassibi.

For my daughter,
Sasharina Kate Hoffman,
in gratitude and joy.

Contents

Preface

Twenty years ago I attended a party at which a numerologist offered to analyze my name. After performing what appeared to be complicated mathematical computations she told me my number was eleven—a "power number"—then looked at me quizzically.

"How strange," she said. "This is the first time I have ever seen this."

"What is it?" I asked, genuinely concerned.

"Your numbers tell me that you make money from war."

I met her gaze steadily as I replied, "I do."

AS AN ONLY CHILD growing up in 1950s Philadelphia, I occupied myself with warrior fantasies. My imagination soared with visions of knights, kings, and queens who populated the English history books I would get from the library. The dramatic tales of battles driven by focused energy and heightened danger excited me. It wasn't conquest I was after; it was the warriors' extraordinary sense of mission. I was moved by an empathic connection with the vulnerable and oppressed. I wanted to challenge a great evil power, to lead troops into battle for the most noble of causes.

Unfortunately, the world in which I was living allowed for few grand heroics. Rather than a battleground, it was a special kind of wasteland. I grew up at a time when one's worth and acceptance as a female were measured by the width of a crinoline skirt, when French kissing branded you a sexual outlaw, and when little girls' dreams revolved around their weddings and lessons learned from watching *Queen for a Day*'s ritual of "improving" one's life with domestic conveniences. It was a vast wilderness of mothers, teachers, and friends encircling me in traditional femininity, creating a suffocating loneliness that I could not name or understand.

I felt powerless to change my fate until Queen Elizabeth I, whose story I discovered at age ten, finally broke that silence. Her survival skills were legendary: her mother was beheaded when she was three and her stepmother executed when she was nine; she was sexually molested at fifteen; and she spent two months imprisoned in the tower, a hair's breadth away from execution herself. She learned to carefully scan the political and emotional landscape for signs of potential danger.

She ruled sixteenth-century England by herself, refusing to marry or to bear children. The androgynous strategies of this woman who wanted to be "both king and queen of England" were unheard of for a female monarch of her time.

I kept the lessons I learned from Elizabeth close to my heart and my head when I broke free from Philadelphia and came of age in New York City in the 1960s. The time was ripe to pick up her gauntlet and challenge women's traditional roles. I became a child of one of the greatest social revolutions in history, at a time when it became politically possible for women to legally gain and exercise reproductive choice—the power of life and death. A time when the right to choose became the fundamental premise of the movement for women's liberation, and when the expression of that truth was every woman's entitlement. After years spent feeling I should have been born in some earlier, more romantic age, I have come to realize that my life's work would not have been possible in any other era but this one.

In 1971, two years before *Roe v. Wade*, I opened one of the first legal abortion clinics in the country and thrust myself into a world that came with battles to fight (replete with invasions, death threats, and killings), opportunities for courage and heroism, and the necessity for bold leadership, strategic thinking, philosophical debate, and entrepreneurial skill. There were barbarians at the gate, self-identified as Right to Lifers (anti-choicers, or "antis," as I call them throughout this book), waving pictures of bloody fetuses and sometimes hiding bombs or guns under their coats. My sword was a six-foot coat hanger held high over my head as I declared my sisters would never return to back-alley butchery. I raised a bullhorn to rally fellow soldiers, decrying the clinic violence that swept the nation. This was my historic stage. It was a war, and I finally felt I was living my destiny.

I HELPED MIDWIFE an era in which women came closer to sexual autonomy and freedom than ever before in history. The very idea that women could rise up and act in their own best interest electrified men and women alike during those years, and the foundational works of second-wave feminists inspired millions of my peers. But my feminism didn't come from books or theoretical discussions. It came in the shape of individual women presenting themselves for services each day. I began to understand the core principle of feminism as I held the hands of thousands of women during their most powerful and vulnerable moment: their abortions.

I wasn't immune to the physicality of abortion, the blood, tissue, and observable body parts. My political and moral judgments on the nature of abortion evolved throughout the years, but I quickly came to realize that those who deliver abortion services have not only the power to give women control over their bodies and lives, but also the power—and the responsibility—of taking life in order to do that. Indeed, acknowledgment of that truth is the foundation for all the political and personal work necessary to maintain women's reproductive freedom.

MY STORY IS THE STORY of women's struggle for freedom and equality in the twentieth century, but it is also a personal story of obstacles, survival, and triumphs. Like Elizabeth, I did not want to give birth to my successor. I never dreamed of being a mother, nursing a child, shaping a young life. I wanted—*needed*—to give birth to myself. And, in the arms of the women's movement, my delivery was aggressive, even violent, with pressures pushing down on me from every direction at times, crushing and battering me as I reached for the freedom to become. Most painful of all were my terrifying glimpses of the all-encompassing sense of being alone. Whatever one can say glowingly about the women's liberation movement and our "collective problems requiring collective solutions," this fact cannot be denied: becoming is nothing if not a solo journey. Yet my singular voyage has been enriched with allies, friends, lovers, and family, unexpected intimacies that bear meaning, depth, purpose, and joy.

Thomas Merton taught that there were three vocations:

one to the active life, one to the contemplative, and a third to the mixture of both. This book is the story of my mixed life. I am an activist, a philosopher, a transgressor of boundaries. I strive to live in truth—or, perhaps, truths. I have not escaped this war unscathed; like all women who have gone into battle, I am scarred. But perhaps that is the definition of wisdom. Perhaps our wounds, the crevasses and cracks in our innocence of perception that come as the price of experience, are our marks of understanding.

My Beginnings

*"To guide our own craft, we must be captain, pilot,
engineer; with chart and compass to stand at the wheel. . . .
It matters not whether the solitary voyager is man or woman;
nature, having endowed them equally, leaves them to their
own skill and judgment in the hour of danger, and,
if not equal to the occasion, alike they perish."*
—ELIZABETH CADY STANTON,
"THE SOLITUDE OF SELF"

I have always loved the smell of lilacs. They make me think of love and revolution.

I was six years old when my parents took me on the Staten Island Ferry to meet my aunt Natasha and uncle Vuluga.

We stayed for lunch, and as my parents sat smoking and talking with Vuluga, Natasha took me conspiratorially out into her small garden. She was quite old, with silver hair and light blue eyes. The soft edges of her accent caressed me as she proudly showed me the lilac trees in her garden, telling me she'd had them as a child in Russia.

Even then I was transfixed by the story of her life. In the late eighteen hundreds Natasha and Vuluga were part of the terrorist group Narodnaya Volya (People's Will), best known for multiple attempts and ultimately the successful assassination of Czar Alexander II of Russia. They were caught, tried for treason, and sent to a labor camp in Siberia for life. Somehow, they managed to escape. They made their way across miles of snow-covered Siberian steppes, crossing

Eastern and Western Europe and finally the ocean to settle in Staten Island, New York. The family talked about Natasha and Vuluga in hushed tones of respect and awe. Audacious and courageous, they had put their lives on the line for their ideals.

Before we left, Natasha gave me a sprig of purple flowers from her tree. I clutched it in my small hands on the way home, desperately trying to pick up its magical scent through the overpowering smell of the Hudson River. Natasha and Vuluga remained fixed in my memory.

My relatives were warriors for a cause, but they also fought their own intimate war against cultural expectations. Never married, they lived together by choice at a time when alliances such as those were considered far outside the pale. And in confronting a common enemy, their love was strengthened and deepened.

MY MOTHER'S PARENTS were first cousins. They came from a long line of Russian radicals, musicians, and rabbis. The knowledge of their consanguinity was a cherished family albatross around all of our necks. Explaining to others and to ourselves why so many of us were extraordinarily talented, we would laughingly point to our "incestuous grandparents" as the organizing principle. The uniqueness of my mother's family was a standard of being for me. Iconoclastic, intellectual, artistic, and temperamental, their lives put most other people's in soft focus.

My paternal relatives were no less romantic. It was 1879 when my nineteen-year-old great-grandmother Blume Hoffman plucked up her courage, left her abusive husband in Lithuania, and with three children in tow, moved to London. Her siblings went further, emigrating to the United States to join an uncle who was well established in Leavenworth, Kansas. Blume's brother Dave struck gold in Alaska and begged her to come to the United States, but she had used up her courage and was terrified of crossing the Atlantic. Her son, my grandfather Sam, decided that he would try his luck, and in his early teens he worked his way onto a steamer to the United States, eventually making his fortune in industry.

Wearing diamond studs and cuff links, Sam courted my grandmother Kate, rewarding her beauty by throwing bags of money onto her kitchen table. But I never knew my grandfather when he had money—only after he'd lost it, playing the horses. His nickname for me was "Citation," after the famous Triple Crown winner, because I was always running about. He would sit at home, bitter and depressed, refusing to work because he considered paid employment beneath him. He is unsmiling and uncomfortable in the photos I have kept, like a deposed king mourning his lost empires.

I WAS BORN IN PHILADELPHIA in 1946, on the cusp of what would always be known as the "baby boom" generation. I shared a bedroom with my parents in a two-room apartment on East Tioga Street with my father's mother living down the hall. The bedroom window looked out onto another four-story brick apartment building, rows of which defined our young middle-class neighborhood.

When I was a baby still in my crib, I would watch pigeons roosting on the windowsill. I heard them cooing and clucking while I writhed in pleasure at the touch of my parents' hands oiling me, their lips gently passing over my body. This paradise was lost when I grew old enough to tell my mother that I liked the way Daddy played the drums. The thrusting of my father in intercourse, my mother's body rising up to meet him, must have sounded like rhythmical music to me. But the idea that I had witnessed the primal scene shook them. I was given my own space, my parents self-banished into a foldout bed in the living room, and my acquaintance with solitude began. I don't remember whether or not I missed the comfort of my parents next to me. But the separation was the beginning of a lifetime of aloneness in the form of both retreat and punishment.

Most summers my family would take day trips to Rockaway Beach. One of my mother's six brothers lived there, and we spent many lazy, fun days at the ocean. The highlight of these days was always the moment when my father took me in his arms to the water. He would hold me tightly as I laughed and jumped at the oncoming waves.

We would take winter trips to Florida. Once my father and I were in a pool and he playfully held me underwater, but he held me there too long. I felt I was drowning and had to push against his hand with all my strength so he would let me up to breathe. He let me surface in time, but I never again trusted his judgment or ability to protect me—in the water, in my home, or in my heart.

Even in my dreams, I was alone. My first nightmare went on to recur throughout my childhood. I walk along a beach, barefoot in a light summer dress. The sky is dark and foreboding and the ocean rises beside me in an enormous, pulsating, threatening wave. It is the color of old meat, and the cresting water creates patterns of stark white veins. I keep walking, my bare feet making patterns in the sand as the wave rises high with tension beside me. It never breaks, but the fear of it causes me to wake in the night.

I WAS THE ONE AND ONLY occupant of my mother's womb. She used to show me an old photo of herself at eight months pregnant, vainly telling me, "No one knew I was even pregnant, like you weren't even there." But oh, she so much wanted a daughter, a reincarnation of her own loving mother, who was her protector and ally against her six older brothers, and who died when she was seventeen. And so I became my mother's daughter, sister, mother—and her competition for my father.

Born in 1917, my mother was the youngest of seven children and the only girl. She came of age when not much was expected of girls except to get married and have children; her own mother had left the marital bed after finally giving birth to the little girl she'd always wanted. But my mother inherited a love of music, and a frustrated desire to compete, excel, and perform. She wanted to be on the stage so much that she had one of her brothers convince my grandparents that she could travel with a dance troupe when she was sixteen. "Good girls" did not go on the stage, but her parents finally gave in.

Her dream was short lived. The chorus line finished their contract after two months on the road, so her small taste of freedom and spotlights ended. She went back home to fulfill her biological destiny.

I felt my mother's thwarted ambition, along with her ambivalence. She may never have had the ability to realize her own dreams, but the need to exert influence was there, and when I was born, it was transferred to me. Her ambition for me was so basic a component of our relationship that it influenced my very name. "A star is born—Meryl Holly" reads the first page of the baby scrapbook she made for me. She gave me that middle name because she expected it to be my stage name; she intended to mold me into a performer. I changed my first name to the more powerfully androgynous Merle—French for "blackbird," I later found out—as soon I was old enough to understand the significance.

She was a good mother according to the mores of the time, but as a child, I couldn't bear the degree of power my mother had over me and the lack of wisdom with which she wielded it. She exercised the ultimate power of *no*, withholding her approval and love when it suited her, and more importantly to me, preventing my father from expressing his own love and approval.

We moved to the second floor of a small redbrick two-family house in Northeast Philadelphia when I was six years old. Every night I would wait at the top of the stairs for my father to come home from work, excited to see the top of his fedora hat, which led to his six-foot-two frame, then that invariable smile coming up the stairs to greet me. He would sweep me up in his arms, hold me a foot away, search my face as if seeing it for the first time, and say, "How's my little girl today?"

"I wouldn't do that if I were you," my mother's voice would call from the back end of paradise. "Do you want to know what she did today?" With a slow, well-practiced disengagement, my father would put me back on the ground and walk to the dining room to prepare for dinner.

As the youngest of seven children and the only girl, my mother was forever "Baby Ruthie." My father, needing the security of her dependency, reinforced her immaturity, so that by the time he died she could not write a check or pay a bill. After a child's fashion, she was stubborn, competitive, demanding, and full of rectitude. For this reason it was always she who bore the brunt of my frustration when my will to do what I wanted, when I wanted, how I wanted, was thwarted. I experienced the boundaries of her parental rule as a cruel fortress that I could not escape, and my rage toward her grew as I did.

My father was the parent I always wanted to be with, the one that I most related to and wanted to be special for. Like my mother, any dreams he had for himself had to be deferred and ultimately denied. Because of my grandfather's refusal to work, my father had to leave school at age fourteen, selling balloons in the street to help support the family. His older brother died at twenty-one from a long struggle against rheumatic fever, increasing my father's familial responsibilities even more. The week of my uncle's death there was a funeral workers' strike in New York City. As a result, my father was forced to dig his own brother's grave with the help of a few friends.

Leaving school at an early age prevented my father from achieving personal or professional actualization, but in his youth he dreamed of being a major league baseball player. He was good enough to be sent down to Florida to train in the minors, and eventually made it to the tryouts for the Brooklyn Dodgers. In the end he failed to make the cut. But my father had the Hoffman business gene, and by the time he married my mother, he owned a toy factory. After a fire destroyed the site and inventory, he spent the rest of his life working as a salesman for various companies.

He was an extremely intelligent autodidact with a book of philosophy always by his bedside. We would share the stories of Sherlock Holmes and recite poetry together. He saw the contours of my fantasy life and entered them, while my mother never seemed to have the imagination or the psychological generosity to move enough out of her own reality to enter into mine.

Beneath his gentleness I knew my father dealt with a deep-seated sadness and rage. He had violent nightmares that shook our household. I would wake up to the sounds of his loud wails and my mother running after him, screaming, "Jack, Jack, stop, stop!" Terrified, I'd pull the covers over my head, curl myself into a fetal position, and try to become as small as possible—invisible—so he would not come in and kill me. He never entered my room during those times, but as with the wave in my dream, there was always the fear of it.

My mother told me that it was the memory of digging his brother's grave that haunted him, but I never believed that was all of it. Perhaps he felt it was his own grave he had dug as well—his future, his dreams that went down into the red earth with his older brother.

BOTH OF MY PARENTS were victims of the dreadful silencing that characterized the fifties. The collective socialization was so powerful that it could not be questioned, and my parents' struggle to communicate and express their individual realities mirrored the political context of the time. Their repression was obvious to me even then. Our family had hired an African American woman named Jane to come to the house to clean once a week. As she went about her chores one afternoon, I asked her if she was grateful she hadn't been alive in the eighteen hundreds, when she would have been a slave. My mother gasped with embarrassment, but I felt that as upsetting or surprising as my question might have been for Jane, my parents' inability to even acknowledge that historical reality and how it was shaping the relationship at hand was infinitely worse. Anything they didn't know how to handle was absorbed into the silence.

School offered little relief from my isolation. On Valentine's Day in the second grade I made as many cards as I could and addressed them all to myself, so that when the class went to the Valentine box to collect our love notes, I appeared to be far more popular than I was.

During the solitary hours I spent in my bedroom I created ways to escape the silence through my rich fantasy life. There, I could be free from the boundaries of my physical self, my mother's autocratic injunctions, and my father's withdrawals. There I became queen, king, or knight, able to move and manipulate the world to my way of being. No one could touch me.

This internal world of mine first sprang to life when my father took me to the movies to see *Knights of the Round Table* with Robert Taylor and Ava Gardner in 1954. I sat in the front row throwing kisses at Taylor while my father sat in the back chuckling. Alone in my room, I was Sir Lancelot, resplendent on a white caparisoned horse. I was Elizabeth I, exhorting her troops to fight the Spanish Armada at Tillbury, with the words, "I have the body of a weak and feeble woman, but the stomach of a king." I was Sir Gawain the Pure, searching for the Holy Grail. I stormed the ramparts as Joan of Arc, played by Ingrid Bergman, sword high, shouting, "Now is the time. This is the hour." I rode with Amazon women, hair flowing wildly behind me as I drew my bow to strike. Unlimited by gender, I was Richard III and Henry V, defending their crowns in battle. I would set the scenes in my imagination and speak the lines aloud.

The ancient Greek philosophers said that to "do philosophy" was to practice dying. Our apartment was blocks away from a large Christian cemetery, and whenever I could I would visit the tombstones, imagining the lives lived, trying to capture the reality of death. I had a feeling that I was a changeling, that I didn't really belong to my time, place, or parents. Where were my troops, my courtiers, my enemies? My demons—anxiety and loneliness—became dragons to triumph over and slay.

WHEN I WAS TEN, I discovered another way to break the silence of my childhood: music. It became my crucible, the stage upon which I played out all my competitive and ambitious drives. It was my family's way of measuring intelligence, talent, and excellence.

My cousin Marilyn embodied that excellence. She was the first child of my Uncle Harry, and displayed unusual musical talent from the age of two. She debuted at Carnegie Hall at eleven, and by her early teens she was an internationally famous violinist. When Marilyn played on the radio my parents and I would sit in the living room listening to the performance in rapt attention, my mother usually crying. Marilyn had the power to do that.

Apart from the discipline her music demanded she was a wild child, never expected to conform to normal behavior. When we went out to dinner at a restaurant, she would pick up the food—big pieces of steak or chicken—in her hands and chew on it in total oblivion to the rules of etiquette. No one bothered to correct her because she was a "genius."

I witnessed and absorbed her aura of fame and talent and its accompanying field of exemption. The scene after her concerts was always fascinating. Marilyn would stand in the middle of a glittering group of admirers, smiling tentatively, surrounded by flowers. My father would always bring the largest and most beautiful bouquet. Uncle Harry would come over to us and say something about the fact that Marilyn was very unhappy; she was usually unsatisfied with her performances, and would mull over one passage or another that she felt she had not performed perfectly. Everyone around her praised her, but the only praise or judgment that really mattered was her own. It was a powerful lesson in the ways of the internally directed.

I wanted what Marilyn had. I wanted to be able to do what I wanted when I wanted—to be the measure of all things, as it seemed that she was. So I focused my inchoate ambition and desire for recognition on becoming a great concert artist myself. After many months of asking, crying, and begging for a piano, my parents finally decided to get me an accordion.

I hated that damn squeeze-box; it never felt serious. But I practiced and worked, and in a few months I showed a great deal of natural ability. After my teacher told my mother that it was time for me to get an adult-size accordion, she relented and bought me a piano.

I knew I was very good at it early on. I finally had something special, something that enabled me to stand apart. My mother was not telling the neighbors that I was a genius yet, but I was determined to give her the opportunity. By this time our family had moved to Queens, New York, and after taking lessons there for a couple of years I applied to Chatham Square Music School, a special school to train concert artists. I was twelve when I applied and was accepted.

CHATHAM WAS ON the Lower East Side, and the mix of harsh discipline and Eastern European atmosphere of the school gave me a feeling of being out of time and place when I was there. It was at Chatham that I learned to value criticism and discipline. In the master class only the best students were chosen to play for the maestro, Samuel Chotzinoff. The teachers could compete with each other through the performances of their students. On the day of my first performance, everyone was there: the students who were playing for the class, their parents, and the rest of the school. The atmosphere was tense and expectant as I played the piece I had prepared, the Chopin Waltz in C-sharp minor.

Playing for Chotzinoff took a special kind of courage, as did all of the performances. It took the ability to believe in my own talent and trust my body, trust that my hands would obey me and fly across the keys, that my emotional and psychological states would translate through the music, that the sweat and anxiety would not interfere with the mechanical process of playing, that the dryness in my mouth and the knot in my stomach could be controlled, and most of all, that my playing would be brilliant.

MUSIC WAS A TEST for becoming: for creating, for competing, for seducing, for communicating, for loving, for longing, for greatness and acceptance. While I was studying to be a concert pianist I was also entering my teenage years. I was quite serious about my music, but I soon became aware that my teachers were beginning to look at other places besides my fingers.

I was attractive. My teachers acknowledged it, and I knew the boys at school were attracted to me. I dressed in the style of the times, with a cinch belt, sweater sets, and felt skirts with poodles on them. Everyone wore these things, but not everybody looked the same in them. I enjoyed being sexual, balancing boldness and restraint. The strict conventions of the fifties fostered an atmosphere of anticipation, of going slowly, and I found a strong eroticism in that type of withholding. I discovered a sexual resource I had inherited just from being female: I possessed something that I could exploit, grant, or withhold.

One Friday night in junior high I was invited to a coed party that was hosted by a group of girls from school. Since I was studying to be a concert pianist, my days consisted of getting up, going to school, coming home, and practicing for three or four hours every afternoon. When I was not practicing, I kept to myself and read Nietzsche and George Sand. My bedroom featured posters of Chopin and Liszt, while my classmates peopled theirs with Elvis and other rock stars. I didn't have many friends, but I felt hopeful about the event that night.

It was a costume party, so I wore my mother's catsuit, a one-piece pedal pusher outfit with a black corduroy bottom and a leopard top. We all played spin the bottle and turned off the lights while the girls sat on the boys' laps. It never went beyond necking and light petting, but somehow, by the end of the party, I had a developed a very bad reputation. The story that my top had been zipped all the way down and someone's tongue had been in my mouth—major sexual sins of the time—spread throughout the school. My reality changed overnight from being generally accepted by my peers to being a pariah.

I was filled with a sense of shame for something I had not done. All of a sudden the few friends I had became unfriendly at school and the phone stopped ringing. One day I went to a girlfriend's house and knocked expectantly on the door, but her mother appeared instead. She stood at her half-opened screen door, blocking the view of my friend behind her, and said, "Go home. You are a bad influence. I never want you to have anything to do with my daughter."

I wanted to die as I stood on that stoop. But I turned around, head held high, and walked home, keeping the secret of my shame to myself. At school I was called a tramp, whore, and slut, all the nomenclature of sexual repression. The few friends I had didn't protect me from those rumors. The bold stares, the faces turned away, and the laughter behind hands hurt just as much.

These girls were parroting the traditional female party line that their parents had taught them: there were good girls, and there were bad girls. They were so easily led by this lie that their friendship and love could quickly turn to disdain and shunning. In a way, though, I understood. My own experiences with my parents had taught me how it felt to be powerless in the face of social conventions.

All my life I have been a target for some reason or other. I've turned my ability to handle being singled out into a political attribute. Walking down a hall of people looking at me, knowing what they were thinking, knowing equally that it was not true, and keeping my head up, saying, "I will not show them I care"—it was a painful lesson. It trained me for what I confront now.

I was sixteen when my parents sent me to Indian Hill Music Camp for the summer. Set in the beautiful Berkshires, minutes away from Tanglewood, Indian Hill was a kind of adolescent Arcadia of the 1960s for talented young musicians, performers, and artists. Marjorie Mazia, second wife of Woody Guthrie, taught dance while I was there, and Arlo Guthrie fiddled away under the trees. An internationally famous concert pianist named Daniel Abrams was musical director for the summer.

Danny, as we called him, was my piano instructor. When I played my Chopin Waltz in C-sharp minor during my first lesson with him, he told me it made him cry. There it was again, that emotional power, but now the energy of the music had translated into the realm of the erotic. It was the first time I felt the intensity of my own feelings for another, the sensation of not being able to breathe for the fluttering in my stomach, an unexpected inarticulateness in speech and action when he would sit next to me to explain a phrase, or pace behind me, listening, watching me play.

As musical director for the summer program, he was to conduct the camp orchestra at the end of the season, a showcase of the most talented students at Indian Hill. He decided I should study the Mozart D minor Piano Concerto as my performance piece. I took two or three lessons with him each week and practiced for hours daily. In the afternoons we would sit together in two Adirondack chairs on the beautifully manicured lawn in front of the Victorian house where the campers lived for the summer. He would pick flowers and hand them to me while his wife, who worked in the administrative offices, looked on from her window.

There was never any real contact; we merely touched hands. But the power of our connection was shattering for me, and everyone at camp saw it. My passion for Danny began spilling out, and he felt it, too. He spoke to me of his love, his desire to be with me, Mozart serving as the backdrop to our romance. Was this love or madness?

The strength of my own feelings frightened me. When my parents came up on visiting day I told my father about the relationship. He was furious, and threatened to kill Danny. When he went to report Danny to the camp administrator, I was filled with a mixture of terror and relief. Now I could be safe from the intense feelings that were threatening to overwhelm me.

After my father's outburst, the scandal spilled into the open. It was complicated by accusations from the administration that I was sexually active with a close girlfriend with whom I bunked. We were affectionate with each other, as young girlfriends often are, but our touching was never sexual. Yet for these transgressions I was asked to leave the camp two weeks prior to the end of the season. I refused. I wanted to play the Mozart D minor with the orchestra, and I was not going to give that up. Danny stayed away from me except during rehearsals.

A couple of days after the incident with my father, Danny's wife, Sonia, approached me. We sat in her light brown VW on that dark, rainy afternoon and drove round and round the circular driveway. "He's really not in love with you," Sonia said calmly. "He doesn't want to marry you. You're very young, you're just imagining all this."

I looked at her steadily. "No. Your husband is in love with me. He does want to marry me. But I will not marry him." Nothing she could say would move me from what I knew to be the truth.

At the final concert I played the Mozart D minor—brilliantly, to spite them all—with a cadenza that Danny had written especially for me. The transcendent emotional and sexual eroticism I felt that evening was amazing. Our music was all around me: his conducting, his gaze, my playing. Nothing before or after ever reached that particular romantic height.

It was a long way down after that moment. I entered what would be the first of many depressions throughout my life. I slept a lot, ate little, and felt an overwhelming despair. I had experienced these soaring heights of emotion, accomplishment, and power, only to be brought low by scandal and rumor. It was middle school all over again. It seemed there was no exit for me, no one who could possibly understand. I could not communicate with my parents about my struggles, and I still didn't have many friends in whom I could confide. Having dipped into Freud, I decided I needed to express the imaginative and demonic forces that beset me without the anxiety of being judged. I convinced my parents to take me to a therapist.

I had always been told to restrain my intensity. My teachers had mocked my affairs with history and gazed with gentle irony at my ego ideals. Now my first therapist, Dr. Stanley Rustin, whom I would go on to visit on and off for many years, described me as a "body of exposed nerves." But unlike the others, he did not pathologize my passionate and artistic nature. He taught me to see it as a challenge and a gift. Our weekly sessions became a kind of pit stop for me, an oasis of quietude, reflection, and sympathy. With his help I gained more power over myself and my environment.

AFTER THE SUMMER at Indian Hill, I attended the High School of Music and Art in Manhattan. A young teacher, Jerome Charyn, was substituting for my English literature class. He had a French bohemian look that I loved: longish dark hair parted on the side, a compact body, and languorous eyes. We only had a few minutes of conversation that day. Then I didn't see him for a couple of months.

My classmates and I always ran down the hall from gym class; the gym was on a different floor from the lockers, and it was the only way to make it to the next class on time. One morning I was the first one out the door, as usual, a few feet in front of the rest of the roaring crowd. I glanced to my right into an open classroom door, and there was Jerome Charyn, standing and gesticulating a point to the class.

I stopped dead, overwhelmed by my attraction, and called to him, "Hello . . . Hello . . ." But before he could answer me I was knocked to the ground by the rush of girls behind me. The blow was so forceful that I was taken to the emergency room at Harlem Hospital, where I had to have three stitches.

Before long, Charyn and I began meeting in his apartment, or sometimes at the Cloisters, a good place for assignations. It was quiet there, with the sarcophogi and sculptures of the Saints, the Lady and the Unicorn looking impassively at our twentieth-century lust.

I was learning just how powerful my sexuality could be, but I didn't lose my virginity to Danny or Charyn. No, my first lover was a Chilean concert pianist, Ivan Allehandro Nunez. The announcement that the pianist Vladimir Horowitz was going to play again after a nine-year hiatus created an electrical shock throughout the classical music world, and people were lined up for three days to get tickets. I met Ivan sneaking into Carnegie Hall after we both discovered we were too late to buy tickets. At intermission we ran through the ticket takers and up the stairs to the first box we saw. We caught our breath and looked around at the box's rightful inhabitants: George Balanchine and Jerome Robbins. "Please," I begged, "We are poor students and we have to hear Horowitz!" They appeared to be charmed by our passion. I was invited to sit down, and Ivan stood behind me as I reveled in the scales of the Mephisto Waltz by Liszt. So began my romantic four-month affair with Ivan.

I had slowly learned to equate sex with power, but fear of pregnancy as well as the feeling that I was now vulnerable to rumors made me feel psychologically diminished after having sex. Though my affairs were intense, sex could make me feel as though someone had *had* me. After the trauma of being called a slut as a girl, it seemed to me that "giving yourself" to a man meant losing yourself.

I wanted these men as lovers, but I was competitive with them, too. I felt myself to be just as talented and ambitious as they were, but they had egos that had to be nourished. One lover, an Israeli concert pianist named Amiram Rigai, had me turn pages for him when he recorded his first Gottshalk performance. He also told me in no uncertain terms that when he got home he wanted "dinner on the table, not Chopin on the piano."

I had no desire to be a character in someone else's adventure. I wanted someone to match me, stretching my abilities and emotions. I wanted more than a lover. I wanted an ally.

NINETEEN SIXTY-FIVE was the beginning of huge, hungry changes for me. Riding into the city from Queens on the E train with my father, I told him I had to go to Paris to study piano—that nothing, no one, in the United States was anywhere near what I could find there.

When I graduated the High School of Music and Art my parents gave me a trip to Europe as a present. I stayed with some cousins in England for a bit and then decided to go to Scotland to visit the historical sites associated with Mary Queen of Scots. I traveled to Holyrood Palace and saw the room where her secretary David Rizzio was murdered while holding onto her skirt when she was five months pregnant. I made more pilgrimages to sacred musical relics: Chopin's piano in Mallorca, where he lived with George Sand; Beethoven's piano in Vienna, where he composed the Fifth Symphony; Liszt's, in Budapest. As I put my fingers on the keyboards I felt that somehow I was channeling their energy. I was eighteen, passionately romantic, and greedy for experiences.

Cynthia Colquitt-Craven, a descendant of English aristocracy whom I had met at a local pub while traveling down the Cornish coast, ran a large stable and riding academy. When she invited me to her home for a visit, we became instant friends. I lived in her small stone cottage for eight months, rising at dawn each day to help her feed the horses and muck out the stalls. She taught me to ride and I learned to share her passion for fox hunting.

I jumped five-foot banks, galloped across fields, and tried, like everyone else, to be there at the "kill." Sometimes we'd pass antihunt demonstrators with signs bearing a quotation by Oscar Wilde, calling hunting "the unspeakable in full pursuit of the uneatable." At the time I was too far into the English aristocratic fantasy to relate to the protesters. It would be years before I allowed the cruelty of what we were doing to enter my mind. In the meantime I rode to the hounds à la Tom Jones, in full regalia with a small flask in my jacket for whiskey. At night I sat by the fire sipping brandy with Cynthia and the hunt master, his dogs at my feet after a long day of riding. I learned to play a good game of darts at the local pub and went galloping along the gorgeous beaches of the Cornish coast with Cynthia for pleasure, wild and free.

Cynthia shared my fantasy. Not only was she actually descended from the English Plantagenet kings, but she lived there in her head. We parried back and forth about the most obscure historical facts, quoted Shakespeare and recited Elizabethan poetry, and walked on the bluff where Walter Raleigh had played bowls while the Spanish Armada gathered force. We were sisters and allies in multiple realities. In the years to come, when our lives became so different— I holding the hands of my patients on the operating tables and she always with her horses in Cornwall—that wonderful sense of connection would return every time we talked. With Cynthia I experienced a true sense of trust. It was the first time I'd ever felt that with another woman.

I went to Europe again and again. I studied music in Paris for eight months, living in a room with no windows and surviving on bread and cheese. I attended a bullfight in Madrid, where I caught the ear of a bull thrown to me by a triumphant matador. I lived in Cologne for five months with Walter Kinzel, a German research psychologist whom I met in the lobby of the Americana Hotel. At twenty-two I learned to play backgammon on the QEII from Prince Alexis Obolensky, just before the first international backgammon tournament. He noticed I was traveling alone, and we began a friendship that lasted the duration of our transatlantic crossing.

ALL OF THESE ADVENTURES were self-selected and self-defining. I began to feel that I could make things happen, create realities from the visions in my head.

I came back to the United States when my money ran out and I received news that my father was ill in the hospital. I worked part time, practiced piano, and read constantly. But I couldn't escape the fact that I was back in Kew Gardens, Queens.

It was becoming clear to me that I would not be a great concert artist. It was far too hermetic, and the possibilities of becoming internationally known were few. It seemed to me that entering this world would in fact be like entering a nunnery, practicing five to six hours daily and giving up everything else. And I saw what had happened to my cousin Marilyn, a prodigy who had the opportunity to become a great solo artist. None of that had come together for her.

Most importantly, I had come to the point where playing music no longer filled me up emotionally. It was too loaded with my own subjective demands for excellence and a competitive edge. I could only touch the pure joy of music through listening to others.

Leaving this identity was an existential predicament. I knew it was the right thing to do, but where would I find the greatness I sought? On what set? I knew that any kind of well-travelled path would be death for me. None of the traditional female roles that surrounded me drew me in. I felt I was drowning in everyday life.

PARALLEL TO THE LIFE I was living, another world was coming into being: the women's liberation movement was gathering steam. I felt isolated, cast out, and groundless, and I didn't see myself as part of anything—certainly not the band of angry young women who were calling themselves feminists. I hardly noticed them.

In fact, the war I would come to call my own—the multiple battles for abortion rights—was raging all around me.

Abortion was illegal in the United States, and women were fighting across the country in creative, radical ways for reproductive freedom. The speakouts, rallies, and marches swelling in New York City were paving the way for my entrance into a conflict rich with history and full of meaning, with warriors who exhibited the qualities of courage, creativity, and integrity of purpose that I yearned to find and express in myself.

In my early twenties I knew I had the personal power to attract what I wanted, and I was unafraid to engage it. I had been preparing for battle my whole life. I had no way of knowing that a movement, a history, a war was waiting for me. But I was ready.

The Roads Not Taken

"To be free in an age like ours,
one must be in a position of authority.
That in itself would be enough
to make me ambitious."
—ERNEST RENAN

While the rest of country was enmeshed in the second wave of feminism, the turmoil of the Vietnam War, the deaths of Bobby Kennedy and Dr. King, and the hedonistic chaos of Woodstock, I found I could not be admitted to college because I'd been traveling through Europe instead of taking the SAT. I was going to be a great artist, and that did not require four years of traditional schooling. Internally directed, self-involved, and apolitical, "things of this world" were far less important to me than my commitment to art.

I liked to hang out at the legendary Café Wha and Café Figaro in Greenwich Village, where one could get in touch with the 1968 bohemian ideal. There I would sit with my black capes, black eye makeup, and long, black hair parted down the middle, sipping espressos and observably reading Rimbaud or Baudelaire to attract like-minded friends. I spent my days imagining how I would make history, as I knew for certain I would. As Charlotte Corday said at her trial for the assassination of Marat during the French Revolution, I wanted people to "know that I had lived."

I signed up for a few courses at the Herbert Berghof (Stella Adler) studio of acting with the ambition of becoming a Shakespearean actor, thinking a career in theater could be the way to actualize my desires. But I grew frustrated and realized that I didn't want to be limited by someone else's words. I felt inhibited by my role as the messenger of another's creation; I wanted to be the creator.

Thinking that becoming a painter might give me the opportunity for undiluted self-expression, I signed up for classes at the Art Student League. While I was a student there I managed to do a self-portrait in oil and an abstract watercolor, but this iteration of my artistic self was also short lived. On my way to class one day I walked down Fifty-Seventh Street past Carnegie Hall and noticed my reflection in the glass-encased posters displayed outside. The image of myself as an artist, an introvert hurrying to class with my black portfolio, was jarringly incongruent with my internal reality, and I knew this, too, was not to be.

My search for an appropriate role, a part to play that would suit me, was beginning to oppress me. Feeling lost and alone, I tried to find myself in religion. I'd only been formally exposed to Judaism through a few summer camps and Sunday school sessions, and it hadn't held much interest for me. I later experimented with Catholicism, the Church of Truth, and Christian Science. These experiences helped foster my lifelong search for transcendence, but none of them satisfied my quest for meaning.

I spent most of my time at home, reading. I would drag the covers off my bed and park myself on the living-room couch with a couple of pillows and whatever book my head was in at the time. I was particularly fond of Greek tragedies and existential philosophy. Not that everything I read was of that highest order: Pauline Réage's *Story of O* amazed and excited me, and there was a particular passage in Grace Metalious's *Peyton Place* in which Selena Cross moves her hips "expertly" on the beach that I'd read over and over again as I lounged.

My mother would look at me with disgust as I lay there surrounded by books, which had always been a point of con-. tention. Finally she insisted that I get off the couch and told me to look for a part-time job. I began to leave the house with her each morning, she on her way to work, I with a marked-up newspaper listing of available jobs to go over in my favorite café.

I had no job experience, so I was open to taking what I could get. Almost on a lark I answered a listing for a bathing suit model. The garment center showroom was crowded with other applicants—young, attractive girls who appeared far more familiar with the process. After changing clothes in a small dark room I fought off feelings of vulnerability and managed to parade myself in front of the two men who were choosing. When they asked me to remove my top, I quickly excused myself.

Next I interviewed with an industrial psychologist whose company, Personell Projections, specialized in counseling men looking for a midlife career change. This time the employer's request was slightly less invasive: "Can you type?" After assuring him of my technical ability, I attempted to impress him with my knowledge of psychology. Ignoring my intellectual overtures, he told me that I would not be hired unless I removed my makeup. I decided to take the job.

The psychologist shared an office with a lapsed Jesuit priest whose parents had been killed in a car crash. The resulting emotional trauma led him to leave his order and enter the secular world. As a result of this career change, he now felt free to express his peculiar sexual predilections. One day he called me into his dark office and begged me to open the top button of my blouse so he could just look. It excited me to play with the power he'd handed me—to see his lust, and to feel the throb of my own. I stood in front of him, enjoying his naked, obvious desire, and slowly opened the button.

I worked there for almost nine months until the office closed down. The lapsed priest and the psychologist could not manage to make a successful business venture.

My mother, fed up with waiting for me to find decent employment, began searching the papers herself for job opportunities for me. In a local Queens paper she found an ad for a part-time medical assistant.

"It looks perfect!" she said to me, excitedly showing me the ad. I shrugged, indifferent to what seemed a rather boring job description. But it was close to home, and I would only work two nights per week and Saturday mornings. At least I would have time to pursue my other dreams, whatever they turned out to be.

THE REGO PARK medical office was in a small two-family house with an English-style garden in the tiny front lawn. Rows and rows of identical redbrick two-story houses lined the neighborhood, reminding me of Malvina Reynolds's 1962 song "Little Boxes." I was interviewed by a well-coiffed, perky woman in a white nurse's uniform. She questioned me about my background and showed me around the office, which consisted of a waiting room, an exam room, a consulting room, an X-ray room, and an office in the back where bills and charts were kept.

Part of my job would require taking chest X-rays of patients, and there was a small darkroom to develop the negatives. As the woman toured me through the space she laughingly told me that if the physician, Dr. Gold, ever joined me in the darkroom, it was not to flirt, but because he sometimes needed to assist in the developing process. It was then that she confessed to being Mrs. Gold; she was just helping out until he hired a new assistant.

Next, I had an interview with Dr. Gold himself. He appeared to be impressed by the fact that I was so deeply serious and needed part-time work to help support my studies. I noticed he was extraordinarily handsome. When the interview was over, Mrs. Gold told me she would call in a couple of days to tell me whether or not I had the position.

That evening, my mother took a break from hounding me to get a job. She chattered on about how extremely pleased she was at the idea that I might be working for a doctor—not to mention his office was close to home, and he was Jewish! I was not home a few days later when Mrs. Gold called the house to give me the good news—I had gotten the position—so my mother role-played as me, accepting the offer with much pleasure and confidence.

DR. GOLD WAS A well-established internist who practiced as a primary-care family physician. He knew all his patients' life stories, their problems with their children, their marriage issues and money worries. From the first day we worked together his compassion for them was apparent. When I would tell him that a patient owed money or had walked out after an appointment without paying, he'd smile and say, "Let it be. It's okay. They can't afford it."

As he specialized in internal medicine and diabetes, Dr. Gold's patient population was large and varied. Patients who were survivors of the Holocaust came to him monthly so that he could fill out their medical reparations forms for the German government. I found this extremely disturbing; it seemed they were tacitly accepting the idea that there was a kind of restitution for the Holocaust. But Dr. Gold put pragmatism before politics. They needed the money to buy food and keep roofs over their heads.

An old woman who had suffered terribly in the camps came to the office each month. I recognized the blue tattoo on her forearm as the one shared by my Polish piano teacher and a neighbor who lived near my parents. I stared at the numbers in horrid fascination as Dr. Gold dutifully filled out and signed the woman's German forms.

Then there was the young married man who was diagnosed with lung cancer from the chest X-rays that I had just taken. I was not in the room when Dr. Gold told him he had only a few months to live, but I stood outside the office listening to the muffled voices and the slow sobbing interrupted by long, painful pauses.

Many of Dr. Gold's patients had been seeing him through all stages of their lives. Dr. Gold was the sage, the counselor, the healer. He was the doctor, historically a position of high honor and respect within the Jewish tradition. His was a loving type of paternalism and compassionate practice of power that I came to admire and respect.

It was his hands that first attracted me to him physically. They held a great deal of power, and I never saw him abuse it. I would watch them in focused concentration as he examined the patients, put the stethoscope on their chests, palpated their stomachs, wrote on their charts, and helped them to dress. They conveyed a solid, protective tenderness. Each finger, strong and well formed, gave the impression of a world unto itself. As the weeks passed, I found myself stealing moments to study them.

WITH THE COMING OF SPRING I was delighted to find a flowering lilac tree in the small garden behind the office. Gently, I cut a sprig, found a small glass to use as a vase, and left it for Dr. Gold to find on his desk.

As my respect for him grew I continued to look for creative ways to please him. For the holiday season I built (with the help of a florist friend) a charming winter scene out of paper mache, complete with a small inn, Christmas trees, and a horse and carriage. I imagined that he was enchanted.

At the end of each day, after all the patients had been seen, I would go into Dr. Gold's office, settle in across from his desk, and we'd talk. We discussed everything from politics to philosophy to books we both loved. I found that this man I admired and respected wanted very much to hear my opinions on all sorts of things. I was even more surprised to find that he liked to share himself with me.

He spoke of his time as a Navy medical officer in the Second World War, when he had made the landing in Normandy on one of the first LSTs (amphibious ships designed to deploy troops and tanks directly onto the shore). He told me of his panic and terror when the boat in front of him was blasted out of the water. Fresh corpses lashed against the side of his LST as the men tried to steer their way carefully toward the hell of the German guns on the shore. He returned from the war a pacifist.

He talked about his impoverished childhood on the Lower East Side and how he had struggled to leave it behind. He remained ashamed of his poor, immigrant Jewish upbringing and the anti-Semitism it led him to experience until late in his life. He had gotten himself out of the ghetto physically, but it was still very much a part of who he was.

He also graphically described his experience as a resident at Bellevue Hospital. Victims of self-abortion were so common at Bellevue that the night shift came to be called the "midnight express." Women would start the process by inserting foreign devices into their cervixes at home; when they started to bleed, they came to the emergency room, where physicians would perform a procedure called dilation and curettage, scraping tissue from the uterus—essentially an abortion. Abortion was never openly discussed during my childhood, but I'd heard of a situation like this once before, when I was about ten. I overheard my parents' discussion of a Philadelphia physician whose patient died while he was performing an illegal procedure. To cover for himself, he cut her up in pieces and put her remains down the drain.

Dr. Gold was interested in my history, too. He recognized my intelligence, and when he learned I didn't plan to go to college, he began a gentle, supportive campaign to convince me to apply. After a few months of our talks I agreed to send in an application. I ascribed to the Socratic view that an unexamined life was not worth living, and I thought that studying psychology would give me the chance to continue examining mine. My therapist had connections at NYU and was able to help me register for three nonmatriculating classes. I got all As and was accepted as a full-time student.

I'd report on my classes to Dr. Gold during our talks, and I came to cherish these times as our personal oasis. Thrown together from different worlds and generations, we found a common safe harbor—he from his grinding responsibilities, I from my eternal state of longing and aloneness.

Our time together in the evenings was interrupted by his wife calling to find out exactly when to expect him so she could have dinner on the table. As the office assistant, it was my job to answer the phone. "It's your wife," I would say, forcing indifference as I gradually came to resent her intrusion. But Dr. Gold slowly began to extend the hour, bit by bit, so we would have more time to finish our discussions.

And then the Saturday ritual began. After the morning office hours I would either go out for sandwiches or he would take me to a local diner, where we would have lunch together before he went on his hospital rounds. "You need at least one good meal a week," he would say.

My feelings began to grow beyond admiration and respect. I would imagine his hands gently touching my hair, moving over my face. My work became a way to surround myself with him even when he was absent. One Sunday afternoon I took sheets of EKG results with me to the beach, organizing them in neat piles on my towel and filing them into carefully marked folders while a friend from college lay next to me, tanning in the sun.

I was dating young men at the time, but they bored me. Dr. Gold was powerful, sophisticated, intelligent, handsome, and warm. He was twenty-eight years older than me, and I wanted him to want me.

He started to tease me with double entendres, nuanced sexual asides that I couldn't help but savor and read into. He began looking at me in a slightly different way, and I responded in kind. Being limited to an unattractive white uniform, I managed to accessorize with high black boots and black lingerie that was slightly visible through the fabric. I caught his gazes, though our eyes would never connect directly. We were professional with each other as we worked side by side, but an unspoken attraction was deepening between us.

My second summer working in the office, I planned a trip to Europe with three friends of mine. We would go to Monaco and Italy and drive through the south of France, staying at student hostels along the way.

Dr. Gold and his wife always spent August in Cannes with

two other couples. They stayed at the five-star Carlton Hotel, which was right on the beach and teemed with celebrities and jet-setters. Before we closed the office for the summer, he had told me to come by the hotel while I was in Cannes so that he and his wife could treat me to an exclusive French dinner.

To my inexperienced eyes the Carlton Hotel was a palace. I was overwhelmed with the decor, shops, fashionable people, and ambience of money. When I arrived, I was met by Mrs. Gold, who greeted me warmly. We ate a gourmet dinner at a restaurant high in the mountains overlooking the sparkling lights of the Riviera, and I was invited to join them at the hotel beach the next afternoon. I did, and we sunned ourselves while I desperately tried to concentrate on the Hermann Hesse novel I had brought along. Suddenly Dr. Gold became extremely upset. He was missing $500 in cash that had been in his pocket before lunch. He demanded to see the concierge of the hotel, who advised him to go into town and report it to the police.

Dr. Gold did not speak French, and there were no English-speaking policemen in the station. I spoke French almost fluently, so I volunteered to accompany Dr. Gold into the village and act as his translator. We drove into the picturesque town with its designer shops and cobblestoned streets and found the small police station at the corner of the square. I informed the magistrate of the theft and translated our conversation for Dr. Gold. Now our roles were reversed: I was the expert, assisting Dr. Gold in a new and strange environment. I saw him looking at me with appreciation. The police report was taken down, and after the magistrate assured us of their intention to investigate, we left the station.

Afterwards we had a coffee at one of the small outdoor cafés along the main square. As we sat quietly smoking and drinking, things changed forever between us. We were finally alone together, not in a small office or diner in Queens, but on the French Riviera. Nothing was done, nothing was said. But there in the South of France with Dr. Gold, images of the way our lives could be began taking shape.

One year later, on the last night in his office before he left once again for his August vacation, we became lovers.

DR. GOLD—Marty, as I began to call him—and I had been having an affair for two months when my father began to get chest pains. He was working as a salesman for a company that required him to carry a thirty-pound case. My mother convinced him to make an appointment to see Marty. I developed his chart, took his height, weight, and blood pressure, did an EKG on him, had him undress, and left him alone for the examination. Later in the consultation I stood behind my father when Marty told him that the pains he was having were due to angina. "You're a good candidate for a heart attack," he told my father. "Don't carry that case, it is too heavy for you. You must change your life."

My parents decided to get a second opinion; Marty's honest prognosis and the radical changes he recommended seemed impossible. How does one follow a dictum, "You must change your life," when the life you are living is all that you know?

The second doctor gave my parents the answer they wanted to hear. This time the EKG was normal; the physician did not find anything potentially problematic with my father's health, and he saw no reason why my father could not go on making sales calls with that thirty-pound case.

Two weeks later, I received a call from my uncle early in the morning telling me that my father was very ill and I was needed at home immediately. My heart sank. I rose from the bed that also served as a couch in my first studio apartment in LeFrak City, dressed quickly, and made the twenty-minute drive down Queens Boulevard to my parents' apartment.

I opened the door to find my mother frantically vacuuming back and forth, back and forth over the same small piece of orange carpet in the living room. I recalled that she had also been vacuuming the day we heard on the radio that John F. Kennedy had been killed.

She looked at me with the terror and helplessness that always seemed to be brimming just beneath her surface. Her eyes were unseeing and frantic.

"Mommy," I said.

She kept vacuuming. I walked slowly to her, gently took the machine from her hands, and turned it off.

"I don't know what happened," she said. "They say he is in the hospital—what happened? Do you know what happened?

"Let's call the hospital and find out."

My mother followed me into the small kitchen and I picked up the wall phone. It was early April, and as I looked out the kitchen window at the familiar row houses and trees, it occurred to me that every spring from then on would be different.

I reached the hospital, somewhere in Western Pennsylvania where my father had gone a couple of days earlier on a business trip.

"Who are you calling about please?" asked the voice on the other end of the phone.

"I am Jack Hoffman's daughter," I said, struggling to control my anxiety.

A pause—a time period impossible to measure.

"Oh," the voice said, "I'm terribly sorry, but Mr. Hoffman passed away sometime last night."

I hung up the phone and turned to my mother. "He's dead.

Daddy is dead."

Her white face contorted in pain as she howled in a kind of primal scream.

In that moment we became unequal in grief. I was the one to tell my mother the news, and I was the one to comfort her. That night I slept in my parents' bed, my mother clinging to me desperately, crying for my father.

I had moved out of their house just two weeks before. I was twenty-four years old, struggling to be on my own and to get away from that eternal triangle. My mother came to my apartment a few weeks after my father's death and angrily told me that I was responsible for it. She said I had betrayed him by moving out, that the loss had killed him. Her words cut me deeply. My mother and relatives pressured me to move back in with her, but I resisted the pull of that dark place.

The week of shivah was spent at my parents' apartment. The presentation case my father had carried was still there, and I took it and carried it purposefully toward the garbage chute in the hallway. I was just about to throw the damn thing away when one of my uncles stopped me. He was afraid that if I destroyed it, the company would have to be paid. I was furious, feeling absolutely powerless, unable even to take out my rage upon this black box, this pathetic surrogate.

I was in my parents' bedroom with my mother when Marty walked in to pay his respects. She moved easily into his arms for comfort when he bent to embrace her. I left the apartment with him that afternoon.

Driving down Queens Boulevard I didn't notice the red lights or the blur of moving objects around me. I only knew I was in a safe harbor sitting beside him. He stopped at one of our favorite diners and over a cup of chicken soup told me what a gift it was for my father to have gone so quickly, never conscious of his life slipping away. As a doctor he had seen so many different endings; this was one of the better ones, he assured me. His words were a small comfort in an ocean of pain.

AFTER MY FATHER'S DEATH, there was no money for me to go to NYU. I transferred to Queens College and took on two more part-time jobs in addition to my position in Marty's office to pay for my education. Taking out student loans eased some of the financial burden, but the responsibilities of being on my own and the fact that I was always the oldest student in the class put me on a very different trajectory than my classmates. I rarely had time to involve myself in the social life of the college, so focused was I on my work, studies, and newly found love.

I was always somewhat removed from the collective reality. After the Kent State massacre, Queens College students were conducting sit-ins, protesting from the tops of buildings, and cutting classes to demonstrate. In my Psychology of Personality class, which was held in a large theater-like room, a student boldly walked up to the professor while he was lecturing. Taking the microphone from his hands—"liberating" it, as he declared—he began to order the rest of us to march out of class, to act! Trembling with excited rage, he pointed outside, where students had created a cemetery on the lawn with four stones signifying the students who had been murdered.

Our professor told the class that we could all leave to act on our principles, but we must also understand that principles had consequences; no one who left would receive a grade for the year's course.

There was a pause, and then a great commotion ensued as everyone stood and headed to the door. They filed outside until I was the only one left seated in the room. I believed the professor when he told us there were consequences to actions, and I made the calculation that going to graduate school was more important than joining the group at that moment. I was wrong—I could have joined and lost nothing. The grades for that semester were calculated on a pass/fail system that term, and everyone was given a pass.

The incident left me disgusted with the lack of authenticity of the political activism at Queens, especially after the murders of those students. Rather than holding them accountable for their act, the college administration reinforced the notion that politics was theater—you could engage in it and lose nothing. Only in the United States was radical political action diminished this way. French intellectual history values the consecrated heretic. In the Soviet Union, writers who were viewed as threats to state authority were sent to the gulag. But at Queens College, you could cut classes all you wanted, call it politics, and cruise through your final grade.

The experience taught me the danger of expecting support from people who did not expect to lose anything by their engagement with radical politics but loved to act as if they did. Even then I knew that it is really only when one can get past one's own fear and situationally transcend self-interest that one can gain courage to take risks and perhaps make a difference.

I did get a whiff of real activism—feminist activism—while I was at Queens. Anaïs Nin visited the campus and read to a group of literature and psychology students from her diary. I recall a small, elegant woman with long gray hair tied tightly in a bun, porcelain skin, and bright blue eyes, an icon of a bygone era. Later, Florynce Kennedy spoke about lesbianism and abortion, giving the class one of her famous lines: "If men could get pregnant, abortion would be a sacrament." I was amazed and impressed by her bold language and her strong anti-establishment critique. It was thrilling to hear that kind of unbound language from the podium. Her brand of intellectual engagement was far more compelling to me than empty sit-ins ever were.

THE EXTERNAL POLITICAL WORLD soon began to affect life at Marty's office, too. In November 1970 the *New York Times* reported that "a dramatic liberalization of public attitudes and practices regarding abortions appears to be sweeping the country." The Title X Family Planning program, designed to provide women with access to contraceptive services, supplies, and information, was enacted in 1970 as part of the Public Health Service Act. By 1971 over half the people questioned in opinion polls favored legalizing abortion. Thanks in part to the work of the National Association for Repeal of Abortion Laws (NARAL), lawyers who had previously emphasized the effect of unconstitutionally vague language on medical practitioners began to argue on behalf of women's right to decide when to have a child. Organizations that had been working to reform abortion laws changed their goals, strategies, and often their names to reflect the new movement for repeal of all state abortion statutes.

A referendum in the state of Washington repealed that state's abortion laws, and three more states, including New York, followed suit. In February 1971 the American Bar Association officially supported a woman's right to choose abortion up to the twentieth week of pregnancy, and in December that year the Supreme Court heard the first round of oral arguments in *Roe v. Wade.*

In the two and a half years between July 1970, when New York's new abortion law took effect, and January 1973, when the Supreme Court's *Roe* decision legalized the procedure everywhere, 350,000 women came to New York for an abortion, including 19,000 Floridians; 30,000 each from Michigan, Ohio, and Illinois; and thousands more from Canada. By the end of 1971, 61 percent of the abortions performed in New York were on out-of-state residents.[1]

In the New York medical world, this political and social sea change brought about a flurry of activity among health clinics and private practices that wanted to help meet the new demands for abortions. Referral networks were set up all over the country by the Center for Reproductive and Sexual Health (CRASH), one of the first and largest New York abortion clinics; the Clergy Consultation Center; and representatives of Eastern Women's Center to help women travel to New York to receive services. Cars and limos were sent to meet and greet patients at the airports. Eastern and CRASH "doing" up to three hundred patients a day was not unusual. New York City was soon declared the abortion capital of the nation.

Like others, Marty and his colleague, Dr. Leo Orris, saw the change in New York's abortion law as a historic opportunity. They were both founding physicians of the Health Insurance Plan of Greater New York (HIP), the first not-for-profit HMO founded to provide low-cost comprehensive health services on the East Coast. HIP had twenty-eight medical groups throughout the city, and Marty and Dr. Orris felt strongly that as the major health care provider in New York, HIP should be at the forefront in providing abortions.

They approached the HIP board of directors with a proposal for adding abortion services for patients, but some members of the board—which included union representatives, teachers, politicians, and clergy—were morally and religiously uncomfortable with the radical changes wrought by abortion becoming legal.

The HIP board's solution was to give Marty and Orris permission to create a separate medical office to deliver abortion services to HIP subscribers. HIP doctors in all five boroughs would refer patients who wanted abortions to this new clinic, which would be responsible for hiring the doctors and running the operations. The board was satisfied because HIP was not officially offering abortion services, and those in favor of providing them were satisfied because there was an official HIP referral source to which they could send their patients.

Marty and Orris decided to invest $12,000 each and form a professional partnership. In 1971, on the heels of legalization, they opened Flushing Women's Medical Center, one of the first ambulatory abortion facilities in New York.

MARTY'S NEW PROJECT became the focus of our evening talks. He wanted to find a way to get me involved in Flushing Women's. I had proved myself a skilled assistant, and it was obvious I could be instrumental in creating the clinic. As I had fallen in love with Marty's stories, he was also engaged with my developing narrative. "Young, ambitious classical musician leaves art behind and finds herself a healer and medical pioneer," he said teasingly. He wanted to make me into a star. Just as importantly, the clinic would provide a way for us to keep working together, to have our own world separate from the one he had to share with his wife and family. He told me it would be our project, our space to build and to share.

Marty's vision for our future was exciting, and I loved the idea of continuing to work with him in a more permanent fashion. But the project was appealing on another level as well: indeed, working at the doctor's office had become an outlet for my inchoate drives, an unexpected answer to my long search for meaning.

Marty was a family physician. At that time specialization

had not balkanized medicine, and you could have one doctor for the majority of medical issues that would arise throughout your life. As his assistant I was part of that intimate world by proxy. I was the "nurse," the person with whom patients made their appointments, who called with their lab results, and who gave them their prescriptions. They shared their frustrations with me as I weighed them or wrote their symptoms down in their charts. I reduced their anxiety and softened the edges of their office visits. Patients' joys and tragedies, births and deaths, were played out in the office, and I was an integral part of these milestones. I was part of their healing process, and the affiliative medical power I began to gain suited me.

When Marty officially asked me to join him in helping him run Flushing Women's, I didn't have to think twice. It was the spring of 1971, I was twenty-five years old, and abortion had been legal in New York State for almost one year. It would be another two before the Supreme Court would legalize abortion nationally in *Roe v. Wade*. I would get to keep working with Marty and be on the front lines of an exciting, pioneering new era of medicine. Having left my childhood behind, and longing for a great stage to act upon, I was ready to throw myself into creating new worlds. Now was the time—this was *my* hour.

Patient Power

*"It is the swimmer who first leaps into
the frozen stream who is cut sharpest by the ice;
those who follow him find it broken, and the last find it
gone. It is the men or women who first tread down the path
which the bulk of humanity will ultimately follow, who
must find themselves at last in solitudes
where the silence is deadly.".*
—OLIVE SCHREINER, WOMAN AND LABOR, 1911

Before the legalization of abortion, before the battles, before the word became flesh and translated into thousands and thousands of women lining up for services, abortion had a particular place in hell. The word was whispered, a shared secret knowledge among women, a lurking, beckoning danger approached through necessity. The act was relegated to "back alleys," performed by hacks posing as doctors, well-meaning friends or relatives, and often by women themselves, alone in their bedrooms with their hangers or knitting needles. A small number of fortunate women had access to one of the few "doctors of conscience" and escaped the ordeal unscathed.[2] Whether the procedure ended successfully or in tragedy, illegal abortion was kept in the shadows.

Until it wasn't. In the early seventies what was once only whispered about was now cocktail party conversation, a political discussion point, and the subject of constant media attention.[3]

Radical feminists like the Redstockings helped thrust it into the public eye by holding a speak-out on abortion in New York City. For the first time, women defied law and custom to publicly share stories about their criminal abortions. Some even spoke with paper bags over their heads. "We are the ones that have had the abortions. . . . This is why we're here tonight. . . . We are the only experts," said a women testifying in 1969.

New organizations, alliances, and coalitions seemed to be forming almost daily to fight for and against it. Soon the issue morphed into a political football, a birth control problem, a population control necessity. Abortion inspired a made-for-television movie, pro-choice art exhibits, concerts, T-shirts, and poetry readings.

Before abortion became legal on a national scale, clinics were the outposts of feminist politics, their workers grassroots missionaries who believed that the decision to have an abortion was a question of moral agency, an assertion that the power of the state must stop at one's skin. Several underground feminist abortion providers opened for business with the goal of catapulting their theories into action by offering clean, safe, affordable abortions. Clinics such as the famous Jane Collective and the Feminist Women's Health Center in Los Angeles were run and owned by groups of women activated by the knowledge that illegal abortion providers left women (especially poor women) vulnerable to death and butchery.

Feminism was in the air, and I finally noticed it on the periphery of my consciousness. It was in great part thanks to the ideals and dedication of these feminist activists that abortion was legalized and Flushing Women's was able to open in the first place. But our clinic was not founded on feminist theory or activism. In fact, I started my work in the world of abortion from a very non-theoretical place.

MARTY WAS PROMOTED to medical director of the small HIP group in Queens with whom Flushing Women's would share offices, so the responsibility of running the new abortion clinic fell to me almost immediately. The fact that I had almost no idea what I was doing didn't stop me from diving in headfirst to embrace the challenge. I organized the appointments, created the charts, designed the logo and stationery, and hired the staff.

I remember the first patient I counseled. She had come to us from New Jersey because abortion was still illegal in that state. She came without her husband, but she had a supportive friend whose face betrayed a well of empathetic anxiety.

I was nervous. In this, as in all of my other tasks at the clinic, no one had trained me. What could I say to her? What would she say to me? All my psychology courses flooded into my brain . . . theories, theories, and more theories.

This woman was terrified. She was pregnant and did not want to be. Coming here had required an enormous amount of courage, and now she was in my hands. I was to guide her way. I was to be her bridge, her midwife into the realms of power and responsibility that are so much a part of the abortion decision.

I held her hand tightly in mine as I listened to her nervous staccato breath. I kept her talking to help ease the discomfort of the dilators. I locked her eyes on mine, breathed in rhythm with her, joined with her to the point of personal discomfort. In the end, I do not remember a word of what passed between us. It was strangely irrelevant. But I do remember her face. And I remember her hand, the hand that came to symbolize the intimate, personal connection of one woman helping another, the gravity of forging a natural alliance with that woman and the thousands who followed her.

That understanding was to come to me later—much later. That day there was only that woman, her fear, need, pain, strength, vulnerability, and hand. Every day brought new connections, new discoveries. We held sessions on Tuesdays, Fridays, and Saturday mornings. I always arrived at the clinic early to start setting up the session before the patients arrived. While my classmates spent their Friday nights on dates or at the movies, mine were spent waiting until the last patient had left the recovery room before going home, sometimes as late as eleven at night, and rising again at six o'clock on Saturday mornings to get to the clinic in time for our weekend session.

I knew from my first week on the job that occupying the same space as the HIP doctors was going to be a challenge: they didn't want to share. Flushing Women's had staked out a territorial claim to the HIP group and I immediately had to defend it. The allergist who used the exam rooms during the day seemed to drag out his sessions as long as possible so that our patients had to wait until 7 p.m. for procedures that were supposed to begin at 5 or 6 p.m. Another physician stormed in during an abortion procedure and disdainfully threw the patient's clothes on the floor, ordering us to "get these damned abortion patients out of here." These shocking attempts to make us feel unwelcome ushered me into the world of medical politics, where, I would learn, abortion providers were always shoved to the lowest rung of the ladder. I found ways to create small pockets of care and safety in an inhospitable environment.

After a few months, the New York City Department of Health, which had jurisdiction over all abortion providers in the city, sent in surveyors to review our facilities and practices. Our clinic was relatively small—we were only seeing five or six patients per week at that point, and charging seventy-seven dollars per procedure—but with so many patients traveling from out of state to have abortions, New York took extra care to inspect every single facility. Flushing Women's was sterile and safe, but the inspectors took note of our meager six hundred square feet of negotiated space. I watched their faces tighten when they noticed the cots in the hallways.

Never having experienced anyone questioning his medical or operational judgment, Marty found their presence to be an intrusion and a violation of his privacy rights as a physician. He was arrogant. He hadn't yet realized that his doctor-as-god armor was penetrated the moment he took on abortion.

We could have listened to the critiques of the Department of Health respectfully and asked for time to work it out, but the inspection quickly deteriorated into a power struggle between Marty and the surveyors. A week after their visit, we received a long list of deficiencies. We were informed that our clinic would be closed down until they were corrected. Marty was furious. "Who the hell are these civil servants to tell me what to do?" he ranted. He felt that the report was unfair, and that keeping the clinic open might not be worth the hassle.

Not having a doctor's ego to defend, I wholly disagreed. Close Flushing Women's down? We'd just gotten started! Here was the first real challenge to the survival of this nascent project that I was beginning to call my own. I was already too invested to give up so quickly. The Department of Health's survey was simply a report card we had failed. I was a good student; I was determined to get an A.

I read the Department of Health's report until I had it memorized, then made an appointment with Dr. Jean Pakter, the head of the Department of Health, to discuss solutions. I wanted to understand exactly how I was expected to correct the deficiencies. She was responsive to my earnest questions and obvious determination to fully meet the requirements.

During the four months that Flushing Women's was closed, Marty was again promoted to the position of medical director of a larger HIP group on Kissena Boulevard—one whose physical space, I pointed out to him, answered the environmental deficiencies in the Department of Health report. Marty would be too busy with his new responsibilities to devote much time to Flushing Women's, but I convinced him that under my direction the clinic could rent basement space at this new medical group and work on getting appropriate staffing, beds, and medical equipment to address our programmatic weaknesses. Most importantly, we could reopen.

After moving to Kissena Boulevard and working out a plan of correction, we were once again inspected by the Department of Health. This time, we passed.

I WAS STILL going to school and taking classes between clinic days. I had graduated from Queens College Phi Beta Kappa and entered a graduate program in social psychology at the City University of New York Graduate Center. In college I had been distanced from my peers by my age and personality; in graduate school I was distanced from the other students due to the fact that my time outside of school was spent operating an abortion clinic. It didn't bother me, though. I wasn't in school to make friends.

I encountered a hurdle early on in the program: I failed a statistics class. I went to the chair of the department requesting permission to retake it later in the curriculum, but he refused to give me any leeway. Not having any real option of another PhD program, and thinking that I was destined to fail, I decided to resign from the doctoral program. With a great deal of sadness and anxiety I carried my resignation letter with me to give to the chair of the department. When I got off the elevator on the eighth floor, Dr. Stanley Milgram, the star professor of the PhD social psychology program, was there waiting in the director's office. Somehow he had gotten word that I was coming to see the director with my resignation, and even though he was not a professor of any of my classes, he decided to get involved. Sitting conspiratorially opposite me, he shared that he had also had difficulties with institutions, having been initially rejected from Harvard's doctoral program. Then he leaned forward and whispered, "I have a secret to tell you: I also failed statistics." As I laughed in amazement at his revelation he went on to say, "All the really creative people have trouble with math." After we spoke, I tore up my resignation and decided to go to summer school to finally master statistics.

I viewed Flushing Women's as an extremely interesting project, a world I was creating with Marty, but I did not see it as a life's work. It was not a profession, it was not a skill, it had no name or institutional reality, no well-worn steps of ambition. I'd always imagined a life of music, psychology, philosophy, disciplines with thousands of years of history and structure. And here I was in an untraveled medical landscape that had only just come into being.

Yet even after Milgram's encouragement to persevere, the theories and critical texts with which I was engaged at school were failing to hold my interest. I completed the course work for my doctorate in psychology, but I lost momentum before writing my dissertation.

I applied to a few law schools and was accepted by Fordham and Adelphi. Law would be straightforward, lucrative, and impressive. I went to my uncle Louie, a lawyer, for advice. He laughed in my face, telling me that a woman could never amount to anything in the law and how he would love to have his son, also an attorney, "wipe the floor with me" in a courtroom. Of course I knew he was wrong—if I wanted to, I could be an excellent attorney—but the conversation left me disgusted. I tried to picture myself as a lawyer, but the truth was, the advocates and attorneys I met in my reading were usually tools of the state attempting to bring down my heroines. They were always on the wrong side.

As part of my psychology studies I had done an internship at the Creedmoor State Mental Institution. I'd seen a little boy banging his head against the wall, another playing with feces. A staff member pointed to a child and told me she had never spoken a word. All I could do was observe them, my power confined to the limited interactions I could have with the children as a student.

I contrasted that to my role at Flushing Women's, where I would stay with each patient through her abortion, taking the rings off my hands and putting them in my lab coat pocket to avoid the pressure of their desperate, clutching fingers. I would see the patients again when they came back for their follow-up exams. I knew most of them by name.

A fifteen-year-old patient I had recently counseled had been terrified of telling her mother she was pregnant. I'd spent almost two hours with the mother trying to help her connect to her daughter, to break through her anger, until finally she began to cry in front of me, saying, "I had her when I was fourteen. I just don't want her to go through what I went through."

When it came time to pay the tuition for my first semester of law school, I realized I could not leave the clinic, not for law. Not, I knew, for anything. Flushing Women's had become a living organism, almost a part of me. Leaving now would be tantamount to abandonment.

AFTER THAT, I stepped into my self-appointed role as executive director of Flushing Women's without looking back. I signed up for night classes to learn business, management, and finance skills. I learned about gynecology and abortion, set nursing schedules, met with city and state representatives, and argued with the doctors at the HIP group who harassed me with their anti-abortion sentiments.

I was in charge of a staff that included a full-time front desk receptionist, two counselors, two doctors who worked on a case-by-case basis, and three part-time registered nurses and licensed practical nurses. To many of the employees, I was the symbol of a radically changed world. I was young, I was a woman, and I had no medical training. The idea of a person like me running a clinic turned their concept of the medical world on its head.

By the age of twenty-six I was hiring and firing physicians. Much to their chagrin I "auditioned" my doctors, staying in the operating room while they performed abortions so I could assess their interactional skills with the patients. The doctors cared about their patients' well-being, but they resented my position of power. They were comfortable with women as nurses, handmaids in the surgical suite, but the very idea of a young woman telling doctors how to handle patients, influencing their financial lives and time, was anathema. They could not get used to being under my jurisdiction, and when there were conflicts they would appeal to Marty. As a fellow member of that elite male club, he was able to smooth their ruffled feathers. He never allowed them to undermine me, though. He made sure they knew that my administrative directions were to be followed.

The nurses and counselors posed a different kind of challenge to my authority. There was no room for me to have my own office, so I set up an executive director's desk amid the nurses' station and recovery cots. I knew I wouldn't be able to run the clinic efficiently unless my staff took me seriously, and since I had no physical area I could use to enforce professional boundaries, I had to firmly demonstrate that even though I was young and inexperienced, I was in charge. But some of them made it clear that they resented my position in the medical hierarchy, their lack of respect palpable with every interaction. They weren't going to accept my authority so easily.

I'd wanted power, and now I had it, but I had no idea how to wield it effectively. I found that the very notion of women having power was difficult for many of my female staff to digest. Many had adopted the popular belief that power in and of itself was oppressive and destructive, regardless of who had it. Others thought women in positions of authority should use their power differently from men. When I conducted interviews for new employees, I asked each candidate how she felt about the concept of power. Extraordinarily, each and every one of the applicants, even those for supervisory positions, said almost the same thing: "I don't want to have power over others, I want to empower others." I would run up against this particular female hesitation about power for years to come.

A few of my staff, wanting to employ the egalitarian concepts of the times, told me they felt that the clinic's atmosphere was too traditionally medical, and that the white coats might be off-putting to patients. We were all equal, so why did medical personnel have to differentiate themselves by their dress? I decided to conduct a pilot study on the issue to put their ideas to the test. I made up a questionnaire that I gave to patients asking about their attitudes on medical uniforms. The results were significantly skewed toward a preference for professional dress in white coats. Patients needed to feel safe, and the traditional white coats helped them to do so. In a world where most women were afraid that having an abortion could kill them, many had never been to a gynecologist, and there were no sexual education classes to teach people how their bodies worked, power—the power that came with knowledge, expertise, and experience—was something to embrace, not reject.

Still, my employees expected me to embody all the alternative superior qualities that women with power would ideally have: sensitivity, openness, and leniency. Wanting to be liked, I decided to try to meet their expectations. Perhaps that would earn me their respect.

I took them to dinner, listened when they confided in me about their personal relationships, helped them to analyze their dreams, and offered sympathy when they spoke of their stress levels. If people needed extra time, they got it. If someone was late, I often overlooked it. Every decision was individually negotiated. Never feeling quite satisfied, my employees began expecting more and more from me on a personal level. I felt guilty when I could not grant a specific request, and this general empathizing led to my feeling more and more responsible for their happiness.

Worse, this method of apologetic supervision put a damper on my ability to make across-the-board management decisions. When I had to give unpopular directives, I was met with passive-aggressive attempts to undermine my position of power. I would walk through the hallways and hear whispers in my wake. One day at lunch, I found a dirty speculum in my soup. I'd gotten caught up in the tension between wanting to be liked and needing to be respected, and the situation was beginning to snowball out of my control.

The HIP group with whom Flushing Women's shared space was unionized by 1199, an extremely powerful institution whose representatives sat on the board of HIP. Mingling with the HIP employees, my staff decided they wanted to unionize, too. My office manager, a middle-aged woman who had particular difficulty with my authority, contacted 1199 as a self-appointed leader of eight people, and I soon received official notification that Flushing Women's was in the process of being unionized. Within days of the announcement, a union meeting was held at the clinic in the room where both the patients' beds and my desk were located.

With that, my attitude toward my employees changed. I experienced their alliance with the union leaders as a direct invasion of hostile forces. Who were these people interfering with my staff? Why was I now being censored in my interactions? How dare they interfere with the way I ran my clinic? I felt a diminution in my power, and it frustrated and enraged me. Since I was not allowed to attend the meeting, I stood outside of the room like a kid at her parents' bedroom door and listened to the rhetoric. The leader used fiery, fighting words:

"If *she* does not want to give you these benefits, then *we* will close this place down! If you don't like what *she* is doing, *we* will take care of it!"

It sounded like a street rally against an oppressive ruler. Regardless of my emotional reaction, it soon became clear that there was only one thing I could do to survive this challenge: submit to the process.

The union was voted in, and I was now in a position to negotiate an employment contract with union representatives. I came face to face with the philosophy of unionization and the way it was practiced at 1199. They used a boilerplate contract developed to suit a large insurance company with thousands of employees instead of one designed for a small business like ours. When Ed Bragg, the representative from

1199, advised me to terminate someone so that he could drive the salaries of others higher, I realized that the union's philosophies did not necessarily translate into better conditions for the workers. Merit? There was no real way to address it, because all raises were built into the contract language. But this was what my staff wanted, and we all had to bear the consequences.

The workplace atmosphere became stilted and tense. These people were no longer my coworkers, but my adversaries. We had to function as a team together to deliver an extremely sensitive service to patients, yet we had no camaraderie. And because I was aware that I could be charged with union busting if I so much as discussed the unionization issues with my staff, I was relegated to dealing with them through the intermediary of a union delegate.

I developed a new strategy: I worked by the book. There were no more decisions to make concerning staff's sick days and personal days and emotional troubles; almost every potential situation was spelled out by contract. No longer could someone appeal to my sensitivity or "feminism," a word employees used as a tool against me when they didn't agree with my final decisions. Staff began to feel that I was too autocratic, that I should be more collaborative. But the union contract had spelled out every part of the manager/employee relationship, and there was little for me to do but follow these directives. Gradually, the employees found that dealing with the union and the details of the contract was impeding their ability to work with me on a personal level in our intimate setting, and that our former situation had been far more advantageous. After about a year, quietly and without my knowledge, the union was voted out.

After that experience I took on a new management style that suited me, one that combined some of my feminist attitudes with the lessons I had learned from the unionization of my employees. I thought of it as a collective autocracy. I listened to everyone's opinions with respect and interest and promoted a good deal of feedback, but I stopped treating my staff as my surrogate family. I kept myself separate. The decision-making role was ultimately mine, because the results of those decisions fell—and still fall—most heavily on my shoulders.

I HAD ANOTHER IDENTITY besides executive director: I was the mistress of a married man, a role I had never intended to play, though I did relish it. Marty and I had successfully created the world he wanted to have together, a world that his family never entered. At Flushing Women's his wife and son receded to hazy impressions in my mind, and it was easy to push aside the fact that his evenings and weekends were spent attending to a home life to which I had no access. My own evenings and weekends were saturated with the anticipation of seeing him at the clinic, which in itself was an enormous pleasure. Our meetings outside the clinic were hidden, riddled with obstacles that heightened the intensity of each stolen moment. I would pray for red lights to lengthen our time together when he drove me home from the office.

At times I felt I was in the Bette Davis film *Now, Voyager*: "Don't let's ask for the moon! We have the stars!" I was satisfied with the stars—content, even pleased, with our situation for the time being, even if I could not have all of him.

My mother slowly began to suspect that something was going on between Marty and me—all those late evenings and lunches on Saturdays—but she never asked me about it directly. One day I finally spoke frankly about my affair. The first thing that she said was, "You know, he will never leave his wife for you."

I answered with earnest disdain, "Oh mother, I don't want him to!"

Being a married woman had never entered into my fantasies; the passion and transgression of being a mistress seemed so much more alluring. After all, I was the one for whom he was risking his marriage. I was the one he wanted, the one he loved. Obstacles were the fuel to our fire, and his marriage was the constant and immobile obstacle, his wife a psychological paper cutout for me. I was too much in love, too self-involved to have empathy for someone I considered to be powerful, someone denying me happiness. It would be many years before I would come to understand the pain I had a share in causing her.

Like any new lovers, Marty and I did rather reckless things in the grip of our passion. Once, we took a few compromising Polaroid photos of me in the office. The cast-offs were stupidly left in a garbage pail and picked up by another employee, an older married woman who worked the morning sessions and had her own designs on Marty. I received a telephone call telling me that she had the pictures and would send them to his wife; she only wanted to ensure that she would get a raise and have job security.

Marty knew the Brooklyn district attorney, Eugene Gold. He contacted him for help and was advised that I should tape all my conversations with the woman as potential evidence.

As I sat in my studio apartment for hours transcribing these unpleasant discussions, I felt sick with fear that this woman would be able to use her situational power to destroy my authority over the clinic and to separate me from Marty. The issue of shame and scandal was different then. Having a child out of wedlock or an affair with a married man could affect the rest of one's life—it was not an audition for a reality show.

One day I walked into the small waiting room we used for our patients and found her sitting there with a manila envelope on her lap. She had come to intimidate me, and to let me know that time was running out before she would do something with those photos. Our eyes met, and I felt terrified. I thought my entire life would be over. Our relationship would be unmasked, Marty would have to leave me, and I had no idea what his wife would do to us.

Playing for time, I told her I would have to get back to her. I was waiting for the New York district attorney to review my transcripts and advise me on our legal course of action. After the evidence was reviewed, it was determined that although the employee was in fact blackmailing me, the tapes could not be used in any legal fashion.

Marty fired her and warned her not to dare approach us again or she would be criminally liable. She left us alone.

Shaken but immensely relieved that the episode had finally ended, I resolved never to give an employee or coworker the chance to take me down like that again. I would have to learn to watch my back.

This was my first direct involvement with the law and its exquisite nuances. Dealing with lawsuits would come to be almost a second career for me; at times it felt like I was practicing law without a license—and thanks to Marty's connection with Eugene Gold, it was also the first time I got to see the inner workings behind the presentation of political power, the personal strings that could be pulled to achieve a certain outcome.

THESE POWER STRUGGLES and political lessons were important for my coming-of-age as a leader. Without them I would not have been able to build and maintain a successful organization. But simultaneously, almost in spite of myself, I was undergoing a sort of awakening I'd never imagined possible. My entrance into a field that I was also creating was giving me more than a chance to exercise my ambitions. As the volume of patients steadily grew, my political strife with my employees was tempered by a growing awareness that the power and meaning of Flushing Women's extended far beyond my own life and dreams.

Legal abortion had split the world open to the realities of women's lives, laid bare in my counseling rooms. My patients had anxiety levels that matched their relief and dread. They were here, they had made the choice, but there was an accompanying fear of punishment and death. "Can I really do this thing and go on with my life?" they would ask. "I won't be punished—I won't be butchered—I won't die?"

It was that face-to-face connection that so drew me in. After a childhood spent largely alone, my heart was expanding to embrace others. I saw that the politics, the power struggles, the hiring and firing, the hours of work that went into the clinic, were all in the service of these women, my patients. Power, my power, could be channeled to facilitate this good. I was meant to do this. And my life collided and fused with the massive force of the history behind these issues.

There were poor women of every race, many of whom had numerous children. There were patients as young as eleven years old and as old as forty-five, patients who so much wanted to keep the pregnancy but could not, Russian immigrant women with a history of multiple abortions, college students, and middle-class married women who never told their husbands. They all needed my help.

The general ignorance regarding women's bodies, health, and sexuality was astounding. Many patients had never had a gynecological exam. *Our Bodies, Ourselves*—the influential women's health book published by the pioneering feminists at the Boston Women's Health Collective—had not yet been published. The working- and middle-class women I worked with often believed old wives' tales about how one could become pregnant. "Can I get pregnant again after this abortion?" they would ask. "Will I still have sexual feelings?" I kept a plastic model of a uterus on my desk, and I would use real medical instruments to show them how an abortion was done. I wanted women to know what was happening, to gain control over their reproduction. As the months and years flew by, my eyes were opened to how deeply difficult a task this was for my gender.

One morning the Medical Control Board of HIP, led by Dr. Alan Guttmacher (known as the father of Planned Parenthood), made an official visit to Flushing Women's. His mission was to review our protocols and report back to the board on whether HIP should continue to refer patients to our clinic. Marty and I had decided to have the clinic licensed, and the Medical Control Board wanted this stamp of approval. Becoming a licensed facility meant that we were regulated and inspected by both the City and State of New York, and there were pages and pages of requirements ranging from exactly how many square feet a hallway could be to how many nurses had to be in the recovery rooms.

Dr. Guttmacher was as impressive as his résumé, and I was nervous about how the day would go. But as we conversed, he said something that so shocked me I forgot my performance anxiety. After observing a couple of abortions he asked me whether or not we inserted IUDs immediately after the abortion. Thinking his question strange, I told him we did not. It was necessary to wait a couple of weeks to monitor the bleeding from the abortion itself, and to give the woman an opportunity to think about the kind of birth control she wanted to use. Immediately inserting a device that could have its own side effects and that would potentially exacerbate the side effects of the abortion was not good care, so I preferred to wait until the follow-up visit. To this, Guttmacher replied, "You already have them on the table. Why not just insert them? I would do that with all my patients."

During counseling sessions, I got the patients' side of the story. They told me of doctors who purposely enacted procedural delays so by the time they got to the clinic, they were beyond twelve weeks pregnant and could not have an abortion. There were women whose doctors told them it was unnecessary to refit their diaphragms after their last childbirth. I heard of doctors who refused to allow sterilization procedures on any woman unless she was at least twenty-seven years old with two children, doctors who refused to insert the IUD when patients asked for them, doctors who didn't tell their patients that a backup method of birth control is necessary during the first two weeks a woman is on the Pill. Women came to me with pills that were too strong or too weak, diaphragms not properly sized because they were told it was unnecessary, IUDs that had been inserted incorrectly. They came with shame, anxiety, and tangles of questions someone should have answered for them long ago. "Should I go off the Pill and use foam?" they would ask. Or, "I didn't have an orgasm, how can I be pregnant?" The trail of pregnancies caused by doctors' misinformation, ignorance, or carelessness was endless. I began to call this phenomenon iatrogenic pregnancy.

I knew that many doctors had a deep commitment to women and their reproductive health. They had seen first-hand the results of illegal abortion. Most knew that whether abortion was legal or not, women would move heaven and earth to have one if needed, and often lose their lives in the process. Some had a political commitment to the issue and felt that abortion should be an integral part of women's health care. Others saw it as a good way to earn extra money. The stigma that has come to haunt abortion providers had not yet fully materialized, so there was little deadly social drawback to offering abortions as part of their practice. Whatever their reason for getting involved, most doctors who did this work saw abortion services as an integral part of women's reproductive lives.

But sometimes it was the most committed of the physicians who were the most misogynistic—though they never saw it that way themselves. They were just doing what they had been taught, and at that time being a male doctor meant being in charge, in control of the interaction and the procedure. Doctors were members of a brotherhood; their authority, power, and good intentions were never questioned by anyone, including themselves. I began to grasp that many of the good-hearted male doctors supporting the clinic didn't see abortion in the context of a woman's right to control her reproduction, and thus her life. It was more of a way for them to control women's messy, complicated bodies.

Often, the problem started early. Most women were examined by a man before they had intercourse with a man. Even in that time of liberation, women held too much of the shame and fear that the previous generation had felt with regard to their bodies, especially their reproductive systems. Being a woman meant you were immediately pathologized, that control over your body was not in your hands. Menstruation, sex, pregnancy, abortion—everything had to be explained by doctors.

With her doctor, a woman had her first vaginal examination, chose a contraceptive device, was guided in her decision about whether to bear children, how to bear them, how to raise and feed them. Women were completely dependent upon the doctor's knowledge and in a sense forced into a position of trust. All this resulted in women remaining powerless and having things done *to* them rather than *with* them.

And yet, abortion clinics were poised to be platforms for change. This new field of medicine provided the opportunity for a restructuring of power dynamics and a woman-centered approach to medical care. In the early 1970s, many minority and special interest groups were exploring their own histories and asserting their rights. Acknowledging patients as a class with rights and responsibilities seemed to me an appropriate analytical and political vehicle for combating the victimization of female patients by a generally male medical establishment. The most radical aspect of abortion—then legal in just a few states, but soon to be legal nationwide—was the potential for women to turn this situation on its head.

Clinics like Eastern Women's Center and CRASH, the two largest for-profit New York facilities, caught onto this trend and put "chicks up front" to give the impression that their clinics were women-run even though they were actually owned and controlled by male doctors. But at Flushing Women's I implemented policies that would truly put the patients' interests first.

To start, I made sure patients were never left alone with the doctor. A counselor or I stayed with the women throughout the entire procedure, fielding their questions and making them comfortable. I was especially good with hostile patients who would answer a question with, "It's none of your business," or "Who the hell are you to tell me"—the ones who had an innate distrust of authority.

Thinking that casual humor helped relax patients, some doctors would make blatantly sexist remarks. "Come on, you knew how to spread your legs before you got here, you can spread them for the exam," a doctor once chided. Another commanded a patient to keep still, saying, "Keep your back-side on the table—you should know pretty well how to do that by now."

These types of remarks, betrayals of the trust that I had established with the patients, infuriated me. My clinic was supposed be safe from misogyny, not another place where women were attacked at their most vulnerable. When problems occurred, I would speak privately with the doctor involved. If I witnessed an instance of disrespect, I worked to neutralize it.

I realized that restricting the roles of doctors was the realistic way to facilitate productive ties between the established male medical hierarchies and my patient-centered philosophy. Rather than expecting them to consistently provide emotional support for the patients in these intense, anxious situations, I put counselors in charge of educating and psychologically supporting the patients. The doctors had only to perform the procedure, and the support staff took care of the other equally important needs of the patients.

The necessity of these counseling sessions, these safe spaces for patients, was instantly obvious. Women didn't know how to process what was happening to them, how to organize the confusing thoughts they faced. Because this was the first time many of them had been in a room with someone who was totally focused on them, they spilled out so much of themselves: their relationships with their parents, distress over their boyfriends, fears about the future. We helped them articulate to a stranger, something that they had never verbalized—why they did not want to be pregnant. To us, they admitted that they did not want to be mothers; that they wanted, needed, to have an abortion.

Some of my counselors felt it was necessary for an abortion counselor to have had an abortion to be able to relate to patients. In the early seventies, many feminist centers were practicing a form of peer counseling called consciousness-raising; women would meet in small groups to "rap" about their experiences under the assumption that the leader or facilitator of the group should be someone who had experience with the particular demon at hand. Women had previously been isolated from each other, and much importance was placed on being able to relate to one another as individuals who had experienced the same problems. This rationale was also operative in gender differentiation among physicians: some people requested women doctors, thinking that only females could relate to their problems.

There is of course some truth to gender generalizations; after all, a man will never know what it is to put his legs in gynecological stirrups. But to my mind this thinking is too limiting. Doing an abortion is a technical procedure. There is no difference between male and female physicians' ability to dilate a cervix or perform an extraction. In the seventies women had become physicians in a very male-dominated field, and their behavior and attitude could be just as negative as that of men. The power lay in making sure that patients were treated by compassionate people, no matter who performed the actual procedure.

Counselors had the ability to shape each patient's trust, which could be made or broken by the right words or the wrong information—a huge responsibility. In those early days there were no codified narratives, no context to help women process their feelings about having an abortion. It was up to the counselors and me to define new models. I developed a counseling manual to train and teach others as I learned more about what worked. We explained the abortion procedure, answered the patients' questions about sex, pregnancy, and side effects, discussed other options besides abortion, and taught patients about birth control, centering on the three main options available to women at that time: the Pill, diaphragms, and IUDs. I eventually wrote a pamphlet to distribute at each counseling session. It introduced patients to the importance of what I called ESP—effectiveness, safety, and personality—in determining which method to use.

I knew that patients in any doctor's office were usually too intimidated to ask the questions we answered in the counseling rooms. Women were rightly afraid of upsetting or angering their physicians, these men who had life-and-death power over them—a power they would not voluntarily surrender. As Frederick Douglass said, "Power concedes nothing without a demand"; it had to be taken back by the patients. Because I knew how very difficult this could be, I suggested they bring a friend who could be there as a witness, or a tape recorder so that nothing the doctor said would be lost on the patient in her flood of anxiety. I wanted to reduce the amount of iatrogenic pregnancies, to rescue these women from the ignorance and prejudice of their doctors, but I could not be with them for every appointment. Each one of them had to be a warrior on her own.

Immersed in the world of Flushing Women's, balancing my drive for power with my empathic connection and compassion for my patients, I came face to face with the questions abortion forces us to ask about women's reproductive freedom. My anger at what was happening grew. The metaphoric role of physicians as surrogate fathers and deities resulted in them communicating in a kind of code, a language that only the members of the brotherhood spoke and understood. And they were communicating about women. Making decisions for us. I viewed this as a violation of their oath "to do no harm," a betrayal of trust, and ultimately a dangerous situation for women.

Women's health needed a reformation, a *95 Theses* to translate the language of medicine so that women would be able to make choices about their own health. By teaching women about their bodies, by sharing this sacred knowledge, it would be possible to transfer some power to the patient.

Yes, that was it: patients needed their own bill of rights. Doctors needed to know what these rights were, too—and at Flushing Women's, they'd better learn to respect them.

Flushed with frustration after hearing yet another horror story from one of my patients in the counseling room, I arranged for one of the counselors to stay with her while I rushed to my desk and started to write, my anger spilling out into my pen.

Patients have rights:

—The right to question your doctor.
—The right to know the background, affiliation, and training of your physician.
—The right to be advised of the reasons for medicines prescribed for you.
—The right to privacy in your consultations with your doctor and the right of confidentiality of records of your treatment.
—The right to the security and knowledge that the choice of treatments and what happens to your body is up to you.
—The right not to be intimidated by the props of medical power, i.e. fancy offices, big desks, and white coats.
—The right to regard physicians and the medical establishment as a vehicle, a resource for your own health needs.

—The right to know that rarely is there a single, unchanging medical truth. The right to be informed of current medical changes.

—The right to be assertive enough to ask what tests are being performed. Why? What do they cost? What other diagnostic choices do I have?

—The right to be in touch with options that offer divergent or philosophically different theories of treatment than the one that is being offered by your physician.

—The right to see your medical records at any time and the freedom to seek another opinion.

—Above all, the knowledge that the right of choice does exist and should be exercised.

In order to help people visualize this philosophy I created a poster with the image of god (à la Michelangelo's Sistine Chapel) shooting RX thunderbolts from the sky at patients on the ground holding placards with quotations from my Patients' Bill of Rights. I had it replicated and sent to all the HIP medical groups throughout the city. My referral sources, the social workers in the HIP groups, were generally sympathetic to me, and they tacked my posters up in their clinics and offices.

Needless to say, it created quite a scandal. Doctors tore them off the walls.

Marty was challenged at a board meeting as to why these kinds of political propagandistic posters were being posted. Many doctors found it extremely threatening, and the idea that it was mounted by staff without asking permission from the medical administration of the groups was unheard of. It must have appeared to them to be some kind of insurrection.

Marty was bemused by the entire thing. On the one hand he was extremely proud of me, and liked being the enfant terrible by proxy, but on the other, he could not afford to alienate board members. I was allowed to hang posters at Flushing Women's, but I could no longer distribute them to other HIP offices.

Witnessing their outrage, I was ever more certain I'd hit upon something true. The concept of women as consumers of medical care rather than passive recipients of treatment—the awareness that women's holding to traditional relationships with physicians was ultimately destructive to them individually and as a class—led to my formulating and expanding on a philosophy that would soon become a movement. I called it Patient Power.[4]

IN 1973, the historic Supreme Court decision *Roe v. Wade* legalized abortion for the entire country. For the first time, female patients were given equal power in decision making with their physicians for a particular medical procedure.

What I had experienced with Flushing Women's in New York became true on a national level. The legalization of abortion brought women out of the bloodstained back alleys that had been their medical habitats for hundreds of years. It thrust abortion into the traditional American medical system of health care, yet, because of its highly politicized nature, it created an entire health care system of its own—one that was to be the forerunner of new ambulatory care models.

The Supreme Court decision, in essence, initiated the women's health movement as a defined phenomenon. It created a visible, observable, demanding reality: the reality of the female medical consumer. Millions came out to access gynecological and abortion services. The reformation had begun, and women began connecting with each other, sharing the fears, anxieties, and challenges of being a female patient. People were aware of the need for change, and others, particularly certain religious groups, became active in resisting it.

I initially called *Roe v. Wade* the medical Equal Rights Amendment. The law had undeified physicians and required the informed consent of the patient for surgical procedures, making Patient Power real. But as I would come to learn, implementing *Roe v. Wade* did not prevent abortion from being seen as a second-class medical service, or clinics and the doctors who worked in them from becoming pariahs in American society. It would be many years before I would come to see *Roe* as a compromise—before I would see that women still had a long way to go to truly gain control over their reproductive health.

I STILL REMEMBER when the words "patient power" first came to me. For once, *I* was the one on the exam table. I was having a routine gynecological exam, but I was feeling vulnerable and uncomfortable, my legs spread, the paper gown just barely covering my breasts as I breathed deeply in and out. "Just relax and be patient," the doctor said while his gloved finger searched and poked inside me. "Be patient."

What an unbearable request, I thought. I never had much patience as a child, woman, or patient; I never wanted to wait for anything. The word "patient" originally referred to a "sufferer or victim," an older definition that shares meaning with the modern usage of "patience": to "suffer and endure, bearing trials calmly without complaint," to manifest forbearance under provocation. I was beginning to understand that women have always been the ultimate patients in this sense of the word, bearing centuries of injustice as we've waited for equal rights, economic parity, suffrage, freedom from violence, legal abortion. There has always been something else, one more thing to be accomplished, a war to end, an election to win, before the legal, political, and social gaze can be turned toward women.

Battles have been won only when women have refused to keep waiting to be given our turn. Was it patience that gave us the vote, rights of inheritance? If women's freedom is like the phoenix rising from the ashes, always in the process of becoming, it is fueled by a collective and individual impatience that is expressed through righteous anger and political action.

Lying on that table in the doctor's office, where I was expected to be physically and psychologically submissive, I realized that the definition of patient had to change. If I wanted to have mastery over my medical decisions and my reproductive health, and bestow that power to other women too, I would have to reject the notion of patient as victim. I would have to struggle against society's attempts to keep me in my place, dependent on others to decide what was best for me and my body. It became clear to me that it might in fact be possible to have power and be a patient at the same time. Collectively and as individuals, we could attain Patient Power.

No, I was not patient, as a woman or as a patient. And after three years as director of Flushing Women's, I didn't believe any woman should have to be.

BY THEN my days at the clinic had begun to feel a little more routine. We were seeing fifty women a week, and at that time I was still counseling most of them.

I can't remember how many hands I held, how many heads I caressed, how many times I whispered, "It will be all right, just breathe slowly." I saw so much vulnerability: legs spread wide apart; the physician crouched between white, black, thin, heavy, but always trembling, thighs; the tube sucking the fetal life from their bodies. "It'll be over soon, just take one more deep breath"—the last thrust and pull of the catheter—then the gurgle that signaled the end of the abortion. Gynecologists called it the "uterine cry."

Over and over again I witnessed women's invariable relief after their abortion that they were not dead, that god did not strike them down by lightning, that they could walk out of this place not pregnant any more, that their lives had been given back to them. It was the kind of born-again experience that often resulted in promises: I will never do this again. I will always make him wear condoms. I will be more careful next time.

It was the very young girls that moved me most. I felt so much rage against the males who impregnated each child—was it her father, her brother, some young boy with no thought for the consequences? The girls, the women, were duly punished for their part of the sex act. But for the boy or man there was no censure, never was.

At times I was filled with a kind of bitter resignation. I knew that I might see each patient again soon. So many of them were barely more than babies themselves when pregnancy came, unplanned and unwanted. They were innocent and often ignorant, didn't believe they were pregnant until it was too late to deny it, too afraid to ask for help at first. "Maybe it'll go away," they reasoned.

I spent hours counseling husbands, lovers, sisters, and mothers whose fury at their daughters' betrayal needed a kind of salve I couldn't give. "Let her get local anesthesia," they said. "Let her really feel the pain so she knows never to do it again." The daughters' heads lay on my shoulder as I sat on their beds, wiping tears of relief or regret or both, whispering comfort, giving absolution, channeling rage, sharing life.

"I would want to keep this pregnancy, if only . . ." I learned that it is in the "if only" that the reality of abortion resides. It's there in the vast expanse of a lived life—the sum of experience, the pull of attachment, the pain of ambivalence. "If only" is a theme with thousands of variations.

If only I wasn't fourteen.

If only I was married.

If only my husband had another job.

If only I didn't give birth to a baby six months ago.

If only I didn't just get accepted to college.

If only I didn't have such difficult pregnancies.

If only I wasn't in this lousy marriage.

If only I wasn't forty-two.

If only my boyfriend wasn't on drugs.

If only I wasn't on drugs.

If only . . .

I bore witness to each woman's knowledge of holding the power to decide whether or not to allow the life within her to come to term.

The act of abortion positions women at their most powerful, and that is why it is so strongly opposed by many in society. Historically viewed as and conditioned to be passive, dependent creatures, victims of biological circumstance, women often find it difficult to embrace this power over life and death. They fall prey to the assumption, the myth, that they cannot be trusted with it.

Many women came into the counseling room and said, "I'm not like all those other girls in the waiting room; they don't seem upset about it at all; I don't take it as lightly as they do." Or, "I never thought it would happen to me, I never really believed in abortion." They felt guilty about not wanting to be mothers yet, about getting pregnant even when their birth control was what failed them, guilty about not insisting that their men put on condoms—or that they neglected to put in their diaphragms. And sometimes they felt guilty about not feeling guilty. Theirs was a pervasive sense of sin, if not in the biblical sense, then in the personal one of not living up to their own self-image. They felt they should have known better.

But they found a kind of redemption at the clinic, facilitated by counselors and staff who did not devalue, but supported them. Redemption in the form of rescue from an unwanted and unplanned pregnancy, and everything that meant. Redemption in the form of demystification, neutralization, and acceptance.

Abortionomics

"The representation of the world, like the world itself,
is the work of men; they describe it from the point of view which
is theirs and which they confuse with the absolute truth."
—SIMONE DE BEAUVOIR

I remember the moment I became political. It was a rainy Sunday morning, 1976, and I'd allowed myself to stay in bed a little longer than usual. Monotonic radio voices intruded on my sleep . . . something about Henry Hyde and abortion. I sat up in bed, all ears. Republican Congressman Henry Hyde had succeeded in passing legislation that would effectively remove the right to abortion for women on Medicaid.

"If we can't save them all, we can at least save some," Hyde declared, referring to the pregnancies of black, Hispanic, and all politically and socially disenfranchised women who would now be unable to afford abortions. They were Hyde's first strategic target, the opening salvo in his war against women. Because of their collective powerlessness and political vulnerability they made for an especially easy kill.

Hearing that news, my stomach clenched as I thought about the circumstances that brought many of my patients to the clinic, and the systemic inequalities that placed adequate health care out of reach for so many. Those women from whom Henry Hyde would callously cut off abortion rights were people I worked with every day. Many were unemployed, many had several children, most were poor and had nowhere to turn for help. My growing awareness that women's reproductive freedom was precarious—that the passage of *Roe* was also the beginning of a war designed to have it reversed—was transformed into a sense of urgency and purpose that morning. I instinctively knew that my life had changed, that the five years I'd spent providing abortion services had led me to this moment. I recognized that if I wanted to truly advocate for women I'd have to reach out beyond the world of the clinic to the broader, more demanding and dangerous one of political activism.

My immediate impulse was to speak. If people would only see and understand the truth, they would do something to stop it! Ironically enough, my first action was to go through the halls of Queens College, knocking on classroom doors to ask whether I could address the class and hand out leaflets. Surprised professors invited me in and allowed me to distribute my pamphlet on the effects of the Medicaid ruling: how discriminatory it was, how it singled out poor women, minorities, and the young.

"My name is Merle Hoffman and I am here to talk to you about a crisis in reproductive care," I told the students once their professors stepped aside to let me speak. "We must do something at once—poor women are being discriminated against, poor women will die!"

Uncomfortable silence. The students listened attentively, but there was hardly a response, much less the passionate outcry I'd hoped my news would elicit. Finally, a woman spoke up. "But we will always be able to get abortions. We can fly to London or Puerto Rico," she said to nods all around.

Of course. I was speaking to white, middle-class college students. They had their ways of dealing with an unwanted pregnancy if it happened to them, and they didn't care to worry about those with fewer resources.[5]

I encountered a similar attitude when I spoke to the women's group at a local Queens synagogue. They self-identified as women's libbers who had made the *choice* of getting married, giving up their careers, and staying home with their babies. They had the money to fly to those abortion havens if rights were cut off in the US. No coat hangers, bottles, or back alleys for them.

I left, discouraged by their passivity and lack of empathy. In *The Feminine Mystique*, which helped to spark second-wave feminism, Betty Friedan outlined her view that the freedom to become a fully engaged person is personal and achieving a gender-neutral society with no barriers to women's self-fulfillment is political. Her analysis did not go far enough to embrace issues of race and class. This disconnect became increasingly evident as I witnessed the demographic of my patients change after the Hyde Amendment was passed in 1976. In the beginning there had been a great deal of racial and class diversity at Flushing Women's and other abortion clinics; everyone went to them. Even the daughters and wives of public figures and politicians frequently came to clinics for abortions.

The Hyde Amendment changed all that. Because New York was one of only four states that continued to have Medicaid funding for abortion, licensed clinics in our state began to see a large portion of Medicaid patients, mostly lower-middle-class women of color.[6] Middle-class white women didn't want to share facilities with poor minority women, so they found other places to get abortions. Clinics were increasingly thought to be dirty, unsafe facilities, fit only for those who could afford no other option. Gradually, the words "abortion clinic" in New York came to be synonymous with "Medicaid Mill"—a label with all the baggage of stigma, disgust, and racism that continues to this day.

This baggage was compounded by sheer ignorance on the part of middle- and upper-class women who claimed that clinic doctors were not as talented or professional as private gynecologists. As more and more women began to have abortions, there were inevitably unpleasant stories about experiences people had in clinics—long waits, scheduling mix-ups, personality conflicts. These complaints were endemic to any hospital or surgical procedure, but somehow with abortion they became writ large. The politics of abortion were beginning to poison the well of experience.

In fact, many doctors who performed abortions in their private offices were much less experienced than those who did hundreds of abortions each week in clinics. Private doctors had absolutely no regulations, many charging patients more money than the clinics for procedures they weren't experts at conducting. Some doctors victimized illegal immigrant women in particular; since they did not have Social Security numbers, they were ineligible for Medicaid, and were forced to pay exorbitant prices to private providers. And hospitals—unwieldy in terms of space and operational function, incredibly cost prohibitive, and unwilling to deal with abortion politics—were often not feasible alternatives for women of any class.

Licensed facilities like Flushing Women's were the best option for all women, wealthy or poor. We were required to meet hospital standards for care, staff, space, and management procedures, and our doctors were extremely skilled.[7]

The Department of Health conducted routine inspections to ensure that Flushing Women's was meeting all of the promulgated standards and requirements. Each time, they spent two to three days reviewing hundreds of charts, looking at every piece of equipment, examining staffing patterns, and even staying in the ORs to watch procedures. During the exit interviews, when they reviewed their findings with me, I invariably talked with them about combating the "Medicaid Mills" stereotype that led so many to choose private practices and hospitals over clinics. Didn't they have jurisdiction there? Couldn't they do something to educate women about the crisis? Did it even matter if a clinic was better than a doctor's office if few patients knew the difference?

They agreed with me that clinics were the best option for women seeking abortions, but they maintained that educating the public was not the mandate of the Department of Health.

Even some of the pro-choice activists who had fought for legalization felt there was a "dirtiness" about the business, that the providers were stained with blood, as it were. Once I was at Ellie Guggenheim's Sutton Place apartment for a pro-choice fundraiser and I happened to mention second trimester abortions. She widened her eyes and turned up her nose. "You don't *do* those, do you?"

This was the politics of abortion, the bifurcation of the realities of the procedure and the political arm of the movement. The philosophy of the early pro-choice activists had become unmoored from the provision of services. Now the clinics were gaining a pariah status, the doctors were being labeled "abortionists."

Early second-wave feminists upheld reproductive freedom as the very foundation of women's freedom and equality. Yet women's struggle against gender violence had not ended with *Roe*. Their biological and historical inheritance of bloodshed through botched childbirths, illegal abortions, and forced sterilizations continued. Now the Hyde Amendment passed relatively unnoticed. Where was the great outpouring of political anger at this affront to low-income women? Where was the march on Washington? What the now silent pro-choice majority failed to see was that the denial of health care to people who needed it and the stigmatization of abortion clinics and providers would ultimately hurt all women, not just those who were poor and black.

The gap between the women who had abortions and the activists of the pro-choice movement who had made abortion legal had to be closed. The inability to really look at abortion reduced activists' capacity to recognize the depth of this issue. How could they commit to the political passion necessary to fight for reproductive freedom and equality if they'd never been inside a clinic?

I wanted activists to speak with my staff. I wanted them to hear the stories of the eleven-year-olds who were raped by their fathers or uncles, the young women whose promising lives were waylaid by an accident. The physicality of abortion—the reality of the thing itself—made people uncomfortable. It involved pain, blood, anxiety, discomfort, and guilt, and it was easy for even die-hard feminists to hold the issue at arm's length. But if they could only feel the weight of compassion after seeing patient after patient in counseling, holding their hands in the operating rooms—the preteens, the older women, the rainbow of lives that came through the doors, the stunning repetition of the event itself—perhaps they would understand how high the stakes were.

I suppose I was making the assumption that what so motivated me—the reality of abortion—would also inspire them. But their personal radicalization, like mine, had to be motivated from within.

AFTER THE POLITICAL AWAKENING I experienced with the passage of the Hyde Amendment, I became absorbed with finding new ways to right the systemic wrongs that were now so clearly visible to me. I had long been a fixture at HIP meetings and dinners, attending them with Marty in the role of his talented colleague. Armed with the confidence of my growing political energy, I turned my attention to HIP itself and the enormous opportunity it presented.

I was in a position to reach out to potentially thousands of women, thousands beyond those who came to my clinic for abortions. The majority of HIP's subscribers were women making health care decisions for their entire families. If the powers that be refused to educate people, HIP could take on the role. Strategically, it would serve my vision and would also benefit HIP. By presenting itself as an advocate for women's health, HIP would be at the forefront of a changing medical landscape, which would ultimately result in more subscribers; in other words, it was good for business.

At a social dinner with the president of HIP and Marty, I took the opportunity to pitch my program. First of all, why were there no gynecological evening hours? Women worked, and they needed that flexibility. And what about birth control? All HIP gynecological staff should be trained to counsel patients on their options. Finally, I proposed we have a conference with a combination of academic and political speakers and workshops to bring these issues to the forefront.

The potential publicity benefits for HIP were obvious, and a meeting was arranged for me with Julius Horowitz, the head of HIP's public relations department, to begin the planning.

We decided on a combination of heavy-hitting speakers and educational workshops to highlight the themes of women as medical consumers and decision makers within the family and society. New York City mayor Abraham Beame was to be the keynote speaker, introduced by Marty. I would moderate a panel that included Bella Abzug speaking on "Women as Leaders" and Barbara Ehrenreich on the "Current Status of Women." It would be a historic event, an entire conference on women's health—a field that was hardly recognized.

First Bella spoke, in her ubiquitous hat, full throated and powerful, bringing the crowd to its feet. Here, for the first time, was the presence of a woman I wanted to emulate.

Everyone was high on the energy in the room when I took the podium for my speech, "Challenging the Medical Mystique: How Can Consumers Influence the Health Care Delivery System?" HIP physicians, politicians, patients, doctors from all over the country, press, and college students and professors filled the hotel's main ballroom almost five hundred strong. Standing there, looking out over the crowd, feeling all the eyes on me in curiosity and expectation, I was at home. I felt I'd been destined for this reality.[8]

MARTY HAD BEEN SUPPORTIVE of my desire to organize the panel, advising me on logistics and helping me see it through to execution. He saw me as his student, his rising star, and I remember the sight of him beaming proudly from the audience when I stepped down from the podium at the conclusion of my speech. He was moving in powerful political circles and was drawing me into them, too. Everything that I did reflected back on him, and the light was growing to be very powerful. I was not just a midlife crisis, not just a trophy girlfriend, but his protégé.

After the stimulation of putting on the forum and the sublime satisfaction that came with its success, I realized that while I appreciated his professional support, it alone was no longer adequate. I was beginning to lose patience with our affair. Stealing moments in Marty's office upstairs, sneaking off to have lunch dates, pretending to be merely work colleagues at HIP functions—it was all starting to feel stale. On Saturday nights and holidays, his time with his family, I was always in second place, alone. It had taken a couple of years for the glow of the romance to wear off and the reality of the *powerlessness* of my situation to fully hit me, but when it did, the desire—no, the demand—for him to leave his wife became the obsession of our relationship.

Marty also felt the confines of the adulterous cage. We had tumultuous, raging, exhausting arguments about whether he would leave his wife. One weekend he took me to New Orleans, telling his wife he was going to a conference. We stayed at the Royal Sonesta in a suite with rooms overlooking Bourbon Street. There was jazz pouring from every open doorway and dancing in the streets. I whimsically ordered two dozen white roses to put in the bedroom. But the romance quickly wore off, as it was apt to do then, and our lovely evening disintegrated into a screaming match on the street.

He finally had the realization that leaving his wife would mean leaving the prison of a life he no longer wanted. He could start over, show everyone that he was made of more than the small family practice and the constricting family ties that had so long defined him. He could show all the people who'd refused to let him into their WASP schools or country clubs that Marty Gold could have power and influence. And I would be the catalyst of his arrival.

We had our first public coming out as a couple at the annual LaGuardia Dinner Dance, the HIP gala dinner held every year at the Plaza Hotel. Wearing a long, light, thin-strapped black dress, I walked imperiously down the grand staircase in front of all the HIP physicians and board of directors. Someone dropped a plate of hors d'oeuvres when we entered. A couple came over and asked Marty, "Where's Bernice?" I answered for him, "He's not with her anymore. He's living with me." I loved the transgression and the power of that act, even though I suffered from needing the approbation of others.

I learned early in life that there is a heavy price for transgression. Marty had been known as a pillar of the community, a loving family man. Now the wives of his married friends prohibited their husbands from having social communication with him. And I was not a free woman anymore; I was living with a man more than twice my age, and my single friends slowly moved away from me. It was impossible to socialize with my coupled friends, too; Marty had nothing in common with their men, who were so much younger and just starting their careers. As a result, we lived relatively hermetic personal lives.

Our political lives, filled with dinners, parties, and dances, were always quite another matter. There were often formal events in major New York City hotels, and I was always seated with Marty at or near the main table. At one dinner, I met Jimmy Carter and heard him speak seriously about the threat of nuclear annihilation; at another, I chatted with Walter Mondale about health care. During a Bicentennial gathering in 1976 held by Jack Bigel, the top financial and bargaining adviser to many of New York City's most powerful labor unions, Marty and I watched Operation Sail's Parade of Ships on the Hudson from the balcony of his office building overlooking the New York harbor. After speaking with Bigel I overheard him tell someone, "That girl wants a career more than anyone else I know."

Many of the events we attended were surreal, male-run affairs where misogyny and traditional roles were heavily on display. I would always dress very carefully for these occasions, choosing something from my collection of glamorous gowns, aware that it was not only my mind that was being presented. I had fun playing along, bantering with the men and engaging in their discussions.

That changed at a dinner Marty hosted to pitch a new idea for a business venture. Someone had the absurd idea to hand out soft plastic vaginas as party favors. The men passed them around, laughing and fumbling to fill them with dollar bills. Shocked, I made a disparaging remark, got up from the table, and stalked out. At another event, women dressed in bikinis and fur coats performed on roller skates during dessert. I stomped out of that one loudly, too, saying that they were treating women like animals and animals like commodities. Marty and I would have major rows after these scenes. I couldn't believe he sat there and laughed at the disgusting behavior displayed by his colleagues. But to him, it was a joke. Men were men, and I was being a poor sport.

Our happier times were those we spent alone with each other, away from the politics, where we could allow our minds to drift from Flushing Women's and HIP. Marty had finally served his wife with divorce papers, and we planned to marry as soon as it was finalized. Furious, she'd resolved to make this as difficult as possible, and decided to countersue, resulting in a very long, very expensive divorce. But we knew in the end we'd be together, and we were able to let ourselves be almost carefree when we took our weekend excursions to the countryside of New York and Connecticut, exploring romantic country inns, antique shops, and restaurants.

I had always loved the mountains and forests a couple of hours north of Manhattan. One leisurely trip took us across the Bear Mountain Bridge fifty miles outside of the city to Garrison on Hudson, a quaint Revolutionary War-era town.

We decided to purchase a house there, a 1960s, four-thousand-square-foot wooden structure with an indoor pool and a retractable glass roof, on six acres of mountainous land with a pond. Having only $25,000 between us as a result of the divorce settlement, Marty had to borrow $5,000 from my mother for the down payment on the mortgage.

Our home's beauty was internal and quiet. I especially loved the pond, where I put up a large log to sit on, creating a kind of "green study" like the one Dostoyevsky was said to inhabit when he wrote. And there was one more touch that truly made Garrison feel like home: now that I had some land, I could finally act on my lifelong desire for animal companionship. I adopted a cat and two adorable Akita puppies, the first of many animals who would come to live with me there.

And so, alone together at our house in the country, Marty and I continued to explore the contours of our relationship. Life outside the city made our age difference feel more pronounced, and Marty, particularly sensitive to this, made efforts to show me he was still physically and emotionally youthful enough to keep up with me. Thinking back now, our foiled attempts to participate in youthful activities together underscored the fact that ultimately we had few things in common apart from our love. He was operating in another world, an older world where the roles of men and women were clearly delineated, and I was poised to tear down any barrier I encountered. There were dozens of reasons to break off our ties, and dozens of opportunities to do so.

And yet, in his way, Marty was as radically transgressive as I was. We had a core connection that ran true and deep and would prove to be unbreakable. Our continued partnership was in part practical. Flushing Women's was often under attack from hostile forces at HIP who wanted to undermine Marty's power base and close the clinic. I was often the surrogate target for these attacks. Marty had to be the protector, coming to my defense, sometimes to his political detriment.

But Marty's belief in Flushing Women's and the new ideas I brought to the project ultimately trumped his concerns about popularity and politics. He was my ally. It was a revolutionary time in health care and women's rights, and we were on the front lines. The romance of it all still held me fast to our relationship.

THE SUCCESS OF THE Women's Health Forum had left me craving a grander stage. Marty convinced the board that with the right platform I could garner a lot of positive publicity for HIP, and despite our philosophical differences, they were smart enough to see that a young, attractive, intelligent spokesperson for the fresh ideas discussed at the forum would put them on the cutting edge of health care. They set me up with Howard Rubenstein, HIP's public relations guru, with the goal to evolve the concept of Patient Power to the level of a campaign that I could present to the public.

My account representative at Rubenstein's firm wanted to start by booking me on a television talk show about breast cancer. There was just one problem: I knew absolutely nothing about it. I told him I wouldn't do it.

I did, however, begin to read about breast cancer, the rate of which was extremely high on Long Island—very close to the population of women I served at my clinic. A short time later Dr. Gene Thiessen, a well-known breast surgeon, came to see me at Flushing Women's.

This handsome man who looked as though he'd stepped out of a Ralph Lauren photo shoot swept into my office and told me he'd heard about Patient Power. He wondered if I would be interested in collaborating with him on a new program for breast cancer patients. In the seventies, when a suspicious lump was found in a woman's breast she was asked to sign a consent form for a mastectomy before she even knew if her tumor was malignant. She was then placed under general anesthesia for the biopsy, and the questionable mass was sent to the hospital lab while the patient remained asleep on the operating room table. If a malignancy was discovered by the pathologist, the surgeon removed the offending breast. The severity of this protocol obviously frightened women away from going to the doctor for tests. Dr. Thiessen wanted to initiate a project designed to make women more aware of their treatment options and prevent unnecessary mastectomies.

I was impressed. Here was a surgeon who cared about women's psychological well-being and who was trying to find a way to ease their way through the bureaucracy of cancer. Patient Power could surely be beneficial to these women.

I consulted with Dr. Philip Strax, a well-known radiologist who pioneered the use of prophylactic mammography to screen for early breast cancer. He had recently completed his groundbreaking study on thousands of HIP women. After meeting with him to organize a workable program, I founded STOP: the Second Treatment Option Program. Flushing Women's became the first outpatient medical center to biopsy patients under local anesthesia outside of a hospital. Through our program we were able to put a stop to the practice of doing a mastectomy without the patient's consent while she was on the table under anesthesia. It would be decades before this would become routine practice.

Dr. Thiessen later founded the Self Help Action Rap Experience (SHARE), a support group for survivors of breast and ovarian cancer to which I donated meeting space at Flushing Women's. With its focus on peer option counseling, full disclosure, and separating the biopsy from the mastectomy,

SHARE fell within the paradigm of Patient Power that I created for women having abortions.

With the implementation of these programs and the expertise of the Rubenstein agency, media interest in Flushing Women's began to escalate. Everyone was talking about women's health. At first journalists were interested in SHARE and STOP, flooding Flushing Women's with positive press coverage on the tenets of Patient Power. Soon, they became interested in me. It was gratifying to see journalists encouraging people to take the concept of educating women as patients seriously—and exhilarating to find myself becoming a public figure.

MARTY WAS AT the height of his own career as chairman of the HIP Medical Group Council. The other New York abortion providers, male physicians who ran clinics in Manhattan, had more in common with Marty than myself, and our relationship was far too competitive to allow collegial sharing. My isolation was suddenly broken one afternoon in 1976 when I received a packet in the mail from the National Association of Abortion Facilities (NAAF). It contained a questionnaire for abortion providers and an invitation to a national meeting they'd be holding that spring. I devoured NAAF's agenda and long list of invitees. There were so many of us out there—enough to have an association!

Over three hundred representatives from abortion facilities all across the country traveled to Cleveland, Ohio, for a meeting that May. The impetus for the gathering was to adopt a NAAF constitution. Their early literature echoed my own priorities. It seemed that I had finally found my peers.

I listened attentively as the chair called the first order of business, the approval of NAAF's proposed mission statement. I was immediately put off by the first line: "The purpose of this organization is to promote the interests of abortion facilities."

What about the interests of women? I raised my hand and stood with what was the first objection of the organized session, stating that the purpose of the organization should be *to serve the interests of abortion patients.*

It was decided that my statement should be incorporated into the founding documents of NAAF. Later that day, people approached me to say that they'd been thinking the same thing, and they were happy that I was the one who'd had the courage to say it.

After the first day, I had noticed that there appeared to be a geographical distinction among the attendees. Many of the New York and New Jersey providers had been operating since the early seventies, before *Roe.* As licensed facilities we commiserated about the difficulties of regulatory compliance. Many of the "clinics" in other states were in reality unlicensed, private doctor's offices. They tended to be headed by white, male Christians who had their own agendas.

A few months later the time came for the first election of the NAAF board of directors and officers, for which I had been nominated for vice president. But after attending a few meetings, participating in loads of discussions, and hearing the observations of others, I and my East Coast "supporters" came to feel that the organization would be better served if I were its president. A couple of nights before the election I was approached by Mel Cohen, Iggy DeBlasi, and a few others with the idea of challenging the election from the floor. I was conflicted. Of course I wanted to be president, but the notion that this coup could be unsuccessful filled me with anxiety. When they insisted our numbers were strong enough that there was a good chance I'd win, I made the decision to go forward.

I was elected president by just a few votes, but I lost some credibility and gained the resentment of a large part of NAAF. I realized there was not enough widespread support to solidify my power. The political lessons were hard. Mel Cohen had told me before the coup that he expected to be named chair of the Standards Committee if I became president. I easily agreed to the deal, focusing only on ensuring that I would get elected. But now I was forced to come to terms with the fact that the power I had gained was limited by the promises I had made to achieve it.

I shook off the negativity that trailed me after the election and moved forward aggressively, sending out meeting notices, working to form committees, and starting a NAAF publication called *January's Child*. A few months later, NAAF combined with the National Abortion Council (NAC) to become the National Abortion Federation (NAF), of which I was elected the first secretary. By this time, I knew enough to accept my place in the power structure and wait my turn.

MY INVOLVEMENT in these organizations was also my official entry into the world of feminism. Some of those with whom I formed political alliances would go on to become lifelong friends. But as I worked with other members of NAF to write a pamphlet titled "How To Choose an Abortion Facility" using the tenets of Patient Power as a guide, I discovered that many early feminists active in the pro-choice movement had values quite different from mine. They were medical anarchists who wanted to deinstitutionalize abortion entirely, to wrest the power from the male medical establishment into what they called the "Self-Help Movement"—essentially women's health care without doctors. Carol Downer was a leader of the movement, proselytizing self-examination and menstrual extraction (ME)[9] and advocating the idea that women's continuing struggle against male oppression demanded that they find ways to help themselves.

This challenge to male medical authority resonated powerfully with me—in some ways, it aligned with Patient Power—but I ultimately viewed these feminists' thinking as separatist. It would essentially place women in ghettos. Why was it necessary for women to forgo all the clinical and technological advances that were part of the medical research and clinical establishment for protective or political purposes? Why should we adopt minimalist standards as a defense against the medical industrial complex, when we could find a way to incorporate it into our paradigms and use it to our benefit?

They were also ignoring the fact that abortion was acting as a catalyst for the development and growth of ambulatory, or outpatient, care in the United States. According to the Guttmacher Institute, first trimester abortion was and is the safest outpatient procedure that can be performed; fewer than 0.3 percent of abortion patients experience a complication requiring hospitalization. Abortion facilities were modeling a concept of service that combined basic education and informed consent with expert medical technology—treatment modalities that could be used for other surgical procedures like sterilizations, colonoscopies, breast biopsies, and orthopedic procedures. A great deal of minor surgical procedures could be done outside of hospitals at 50 percent of the cost. Abortion was changing medicine.

I did support the movement for trained nurse midwives to perform first trimester abortions, but I wasn't comfortable with the practice of menstrual extractions. Because the MEs were conducted before a woman's pregnancy could be confirmed by a blood or urine test, there was a 50 percent chance that the MEs were entirely unnecessary, potentially resulting in infections. I did not see ME as an innocuous procedure.

The most radical feminists believed that abortion, and all medical procedures, should be free of government involvement and free of cost. This struck me as wildly naive. How did they expect providers to pay for equipment, staff, and doctors? I was charging a minimal amount for the procedure, but I had to charge something. Yet the idea of making money through providing abortions was deeply antithetical to these feminists. Many had a problem with my way of operating, believing it impossible to be a feminist and a capitalist at the same time.

AS I BECAME more involved in defining the pro-choice movement, I grew increasingly aware of much greater challenges than these internal disagreements about how to make abortion available to women. From this vantage point I could see that the movement for women's rights had enjoyed a brief period of public popularity in the early seventies that eventually led to the legalization of abortion and granted us the temporary luxury of debating the finer points of providing abortions. But before women really had the chance to move into their power, the public discussion began to move toward the construction of simplistic, judgmental abortion narratives designed to put women back in their place.

Two sides emerged, as if they were mutually exclusive. There was either the "right to life" or the "right to choose." Women couldn't help but internalize these narrow ways of seeing the issue and themselves accordingly. Abortion *was* a woman's right, both legally, with the passage of *Roe v. Wade*, and as a matter of biology, equality, and justice. But each woman's acceptance of her natural right was challenged and threatened by a Greek chorus screaming "murderer" at her for exercising that power.

This bifurcation was expressed eloquently by a young patient I once had. She was only nineteen years old. It was her first abortion, and she had come alone. "It was such a difficult choice for me to make," she said softly. "The mother in me wanted so much to have it, to love it, to see it grow . . . The other part knew that it was impossible."

The "other part"? For so many women, choosing abortion created this other—the one who would never have chosen this path, the good mother sitting in judgment and separating herself from the one choosing abortion. It was a formula for amplifying guilt and regret.

The growing political debate on abortion in the seventies took this reduction of women's self-identity even further by positioning the woman and fetus as adversaries. There was no way that one could advocate for both; if you believed in the right to life of the fetus, then the woman, by definition, had to come second. And if you believed in a woman's right to choose, the fetus took second place.

The pro-choice movement had to find a way to navigate these narratives. The simplest option was to negate the claims of the opposition. And so many pro-choice advocates claimed the fetus was not alive, and that abortion was not the act of terminating it. They chose to de-personalize the fetus, to see it as amorphous residue, to say that it was "only blood and tissue."

What I saw running through those vacuum tubes when I first started my work *was* only blood and tissue, unformed and messy. It was easy to imagine the fetus as a bunch of cells that one could define as one wished. But even in the beginning I had an inkling that this mentality was the easy way out, that it didn't go far enough to do justice to the experience of abortion.

The anti-choice movement claimed that if women knew what abortion really was, if only the providers had told them the truth, they would never have killed their babies. Organizations such as Women Exploited By Abortion (WEBA) and American Victims of Abortion (AVA) were composed entirely of women who'd had abortions, but had "seen the light" and become anti-choice activists.

But women did know the truth, just as I knew it, deep down, when I allowed myself to recognize it. Mothers saw the sonogram pictures, knew that sound bites assuring them that abortion was no different from any other benign outpatient surgery were false—knew that, as the antis say, "abortion stops a beating heart." They knew that abortion was the termination of potential life.

They knew it, but my patients who made the choice to have an abortion also knew they were making the right one, a decision so vital it was worth stopping that heart. Sometimes they felt a deep sense of the loss of possibility. In the majority of cases, they felt a deep sense of relief and the power that comes from taking responsibility for one's own life.

There is a reason that women have been having abortions, legal or not, for all of history. The act of choosing whether or not to have a child is often an act of love, and always an act of survival. "Choice" is sometimes not a choice at all. It is an outcome determined by the economic, physical, sociological, and political factors that surround women and move them toward the only action that allows them to survive at that point in their lives. Survival can sometimes be a woman's act of staying alive, but it can also be her act of refusing to put what will become an impossible burden on her shoulders.

At times this reality would move me profoundly as I sat opposite the women I counseled prior to their abortions, acutely aware of the potential lives growing inside them that would soon cease to exist. I began to think critically, to come to terms with what was going on. Each time I did that, I came out of that process more committed than before. I had no conception, either religious or philosophical, that "life was sacred."

My bond with my patients grew stronger as I held their hands and watched the blood flow through the tubes into the suction machine. I was aware of fetal existence, the meaning of that blood and tissue. But it never overshadowed the woman. To me, there was never a question about who should survive.

The pro-choice movement marched then, as it does now, under the banner of choice—of human and civil rights—that is always more nuanced than the pure white banner of "innocence" and "life" carried by our opponents. But attempting to simplify the issue, refusing to look at the consequences or true nature of abortion—the blood, the observable parts of the fetus, the irrevocable endings, the power of deciding whether or not to bring a new life into this world—reduces our capacity to register the depth of this issue and disrespects the profound political and social struggle women's choices engender in our society.

Asking women to deny this truth, putting them in a defensive position, also perpetuates the shame, embarrassment, and ambivalence that the antis want women to feel. "*They* have abortions for the wrong reasons. *They* want to look good in bathing suits. *They* want to get their PhDs," the antis have always said. Pro-choicers join in this chorus with sentiments like, "I wouldn't have an abortion if I were married," or "Why did she wait so long, until she was four or five months pregnant? If I were in the same set of circumstances, I would not have made her choice."

But when "they" becomes "me"—when women are faced with the decision personally and choose to have an abortion—they are able to justify their own reasons as sufficient. When I started to notice this phenomenon I named it the "rape, incest, or me" position. It places undue importance on women's reasons for making their choices, leaving room for the argument that abortion is wrong because women's reasons for having abortions are wrong.

This position betrays a lack of commitment to reproductive freedom. When an individual makes a choice, it is the act of making it, the active will and power of the choosing itself, that has unconditional value. At its core, the issue is about separating the chooser from the choice. The woman is the only active agent in this decision-making process—not the state, the court, or any political body. In a world where men have historically defined criminal, ethical, moral, and religious aspects of communal and political life, a woman choosing abortion is exercising her right to decide what happens to her body, her life, and her family.

I remember an exercise given to abortion providers at a conference I attended. "If you had only one abortion left to give," we were asked, "to whom would you give it? A woman with HIV, a twelve-year-old, a forty-eight-year-old, a woman who was raped, a woman who wants to finish her PhD? What about the woman who just doesn't want a baby?" The catch, of course, is that all of these reasons for making the choice to have an abortion are equally valid. *Why* a woman makes a decision to have an abortion is not the deciding issue. She is making the choice that is right for her, and that is what matters.

If the personal is the political, as the feminist slogan goes, then abortion is the ultimate political act. It is not politics, but necessity that drives women's choices, necessity that forms the political and theoretical foundation for the right to choose. To withhold that right for any reason is to deny women a piece of their humanity.

In the late seventies the pro-choice movement faced the same political question it faces today. How can we create a new narrative in which choice and reproductive freedom are the theory, and abortion is the practice? How can we transcend limiting narratives and start to identify with all women struggling to make choices, defending them rather than resisting that power through guilt and denial? How do we create a world where women can have abortions without apology?

IN 1978, after years of operating in the cramped basement where Flushing Women's Medical Center got its start, I realized I needed more space to put Patient Power into practice. I wanted to build a facility that would serve as a model for other clinics around the country—perhaps around the world.

Flushing Women's had grown to service over one hundred patients per week. We had enough financial stability to afford a rent that was not subsidized, agree to a multiyear lease, and assume the responsibilities of the projected costs that would come with designing a new space and hiring additional employees. The hard part was getting the Department of Health's approval for a new location—and of course, convincing Marty and Dr. Orris that the project could succeed on its own terms.

In those years, finding landlords who would agree to rent space to an abortion clinic was not nearly as difficult as it is today. I found a seven-thousand-square-foot commercial space in a large building on Queens Boulevard owned by Samuel LeFrak. Marty was successful in getting HIP to countersign a twenty-year lease on the property, and soon I was ready to design, furnish, and open my own clinic.

My goal was to create the most noninstitutional environment I could imagine. I chose large, comfortable, purple and red chairs where patients could wait with their friends or significant others. The chairs would have been more fitting at a discotheque, but the patients loved them. The counseling rooms were warm and cheerfully decorated, and I chose not to furnish them with desks, to minimize the power differential between patients and providers. The ambulatory patient lounge had a kitchenette where post-surgery refreshments were prepared, and there was a dressing room where the patients could take their time before leaving the clinic. I filled the walls with artwork featuring powerful women, calm landscapes, and political posters.

Inside the examining rooms, patients received navy tailored smocks instead of gappy paper gowns so they would not feel so naked and vulnerable. I had warming trays for the speculums built into the exam tables, knowing that there is nothing quite as shocking and uncomfortable as the invasion of an ice-cold metal speculum.

My new clinic needed a name, something that embodied the spirit of the facility I was endeavoring to create. I held a competition among the staff to choose one. We collectively agreed that the best name would be simple. Choices. Wanting the letters to hold special meaning, I turned it into an acronym: Creative Health Organization for Information Counseling and Educational Services. I designed a logo to go with the name, a combination of the caduceus and the mathematical symbol for infinity, a visual expression of the myriad of medical choices my clinic would offer.

With the opening of its doors, Choices immediately garnered a great deal of favorable press. I became a person of interest and fascination. "What is abortion, really?" people would ask. "How much does it hurt?" "What is wrong with these women?" "Do you really see the fetus?" Choices became a teaching tool, a community space, a place where every question was welcome. A few friends and family members volunteered at the clinic. My mother came in a few times, handing out tea and cookies to patients in the recovery room.

I set up a gynecological and family planning practice and offered IUD insertions, diaphragms, and oral contraceptives. Patients who wanted to keep their pregnancies were welcome to take part in our prenatal program, and we delivered babies at our affiliated hospitals.

Perhaps the most unique aspect of Choices—the change that fully embodied my vision of Patient Power—was the role of counselors. I began calling them facilitators instead, feeling that the word "counselor" implicitly designated that person as having power to change or manipulate the counselee. The word "facilitate" means to assist, to make easier, to guide the way. At Choices patients weren't forced into the passive role of medical victims. My facilitators were trained in family planning and abortion care and they functioned as a support system.

While degrees and credentials are factors in professional ability or expertise, the most important qualities that any individual in the health field can have are empathy, openness, and the ability to create a positive response within another individual—what I came to call "active loving." The sessions at Choices were structured more like warm conversations than anything else. Medical information was given, consents were signed, abortion and other options were discussed, but all in an easy atmosphere where a person felt safe and autonomous till the end of her stay. There was never coercion; the existence of our prenatal program said that louder than any voice could. We facilitated each woman's experience within her own reality.

ON JANUARY 7, 1979 my name was listed in a CUNY insert in the *New York Times* as a distinguished alumnus along with Sylvia Porter, Ruby Dee, Irving Kristol, Bernard Malamud, and two Nobel prize winners: Robert Hofstadter and Rosalyn Yalow. Articles in the *New York Times, Newsday, Women's Week*, the *Star*, and the *New York Daily News* lauded the layout of Choices, the workshops I set up, and my ideas about Patient Power.

But my work was being noticed by others besides feminists and liberal journalists. I remember being in a plane coming back from a pro-choice meeting and learning, as we landed, that there had been demonstrators in front of Choices for the first time. I was amazed, frightened, and enraged; I suppose in some way I'd thought all that positive press would inoculate me, that no one would touch me if the *New York Times* was behind me. But like all abortion providers, I soon found I had as many enemies as I had friends.

Abortion as a Mother's Act

"Freedom is fragile and must be protected. To sacrifice it,
even as a temporary measure, is to betray it."
— GERMAINE GREER

Never one to romanticize marriage, I viewed mine as the spoils of war. On June 30, 1979, after three years of struggling for Marty's divorce to be finalized, we were formally married in New York.

We had a wonderful wedding in Garrison, but even on that night, differences permeated our union. We would always love each other, but our expression of that love began to change, to grow complicated. Ours was not to be anyone's traditional definition of happily ever after. We had our joint empires and our two homes before we were married. We had no plans to move to another location, or buy a new house, or begin having children.

I knew our time was limited and that I was not going to grow old with Marty. The Rubicon had been crossed, and with that came a nagging sense of despair. The battle to be together was replaced over the years by many others, but that was the first, and the dearest, and it was over.

WHAT NOW? I was not the only woman struggling to answer that question; it seemed to be in the air. Now that abortion was legal and women empowered, how would society change? The search for answers brought about a heightened public interest in how abortion functioned in women's lives. A *New York Post* investigation[10] reported that 20 percent of New York women had had an abortion since its legalization in the state almost ten years earlier. Soon after, the Supreme Court ruled that teenage girls need not obtain parental consent in order to have an abortion.[11] Choices and other clinics continued to be publicly lauded for pioneering a new women's health movement. Advocates for women's rights were trying to articulate the path from legalized abortion to a changed society, one in which the expression of female sexuality was truly free from the traditional bonds of reproduction.

The pro-choice movement's prominence in mainstream media and public consciousness was paralleled by the growth of the anti-choice movement, members of which could increasingly be seen demonstrating outside abortion clinics across the country. But the glow of legalization disallowed the idea that there could be a viable political challenge to *Roe* at this early point. Many of my pro-choice colleagues thought the possibility of a return to back alleys was inconceivable. It was hard to take the antis seriously. When Ellie Smeal of the National Organization for Women (NOW) called together pro- and anti-choice contingents for a dialogue in 1979, an anti-choice group held up jars of pickled fetuses and prevented productive discourse. Their oversimplified battle cry, "Don't kill your baby!" seemed almost too easy to defeat, and emboldened by our relatively recent victory, we allowed ourselves to take a well-deserved, collective deep breath.

But we would have to learn that in this war, with this issue, the combatants never have much time to breathe. I was soon forced to thrust my way daily through a throng of protesters who gathered at the entrance of Choices. I knew that our side was in danger of falling prey to the most fundamental strategic failure: underestimating the opposition. The antis were not going away.

Unfortunately, they began proving me right on a massive political scale. In 1979 the American Life League was formed by Roman Catholics Judy and Paul Brown. The ultimate abortion abolitionists, members of this group believed that the procedure was unacceptable even in the case of rape or when a woman's life was endangered. A year later former Catholic seminarian Joseph Scheidler founded the Pro-Life Action League and began to organize abortion clinic invasions. The National Right to Life Committee busily laid the philosophical foundation of the modern right-to-life movement by connecting abortion to euthanasia and assisted suicide, while fundamentalist anti-abortionists produced a Nuremberg-style "hit list" of pro-choice providers to be targeted for harassment or worse.

Anti-choice sentiment blossomed more broadly with the founding and growth of popular televangelist Jerry Falwell's Moral Majority, a hugely influential evangelical lobbying organization with an adamant pro-life agenda. Republicans had always taken a firm position in favor of a constitutional amendment banning abortion, but democrats were also affected by this social and political shift to the right. Jimmy Carter, the first evangelical Christian to become president, famously forsook his party's pro-choice plank when he defended his support for the Hyde Amendment with the statement "Life is unfair"—a lack of commitment to abortion rights that democratic politicians would continue to exhibit, even though the party's official pro-choice stance didn't change.

The possibility that Congress could favor a ban on abortion became more difficult for the pro-choice movement to dismiss. Representative Romano Mazzoli proposed the Paramount Amendment, a "Human Life" bill that would circumvent the long process of passing a constitutional amendment to outlaw abortion by having Congress vote that human life began at conception. With its passage, Congress could trump science and religious differences by co-opting the ultimate authority to define when life begins, then moving aggressively to protect that life by outlawing abortions.

The bill didn't pass, but the idea that such an amendment was even up for discussion infuriated me. A sperm and egg were to equal a person at the moment of conception? A fertilized egg—whether or not it was "alive"—would have the same rights as I would? How could a fetus ever take on the responsibilities of personhood? But I was not in the land of reality among the antis. Logical arguments were met with arrogant dismissal by these true believers. Life was life; fertilized eggs were people who had to be protected, and damn the women whose bodies housed them.

It was a power struggle, pure and simple, the same struggle that continues to this day: Who holds the power to decide whether a fetus should come to term? Who has the power to decide whether a woman should give birth, how many children she should have, what constitutes a "good" mother?

Ironically, the New Right and Moral Majority were as in touch with the fact that abortion empowers women as women's rights activists. The antis clearly understood that to keep women in the traditional roles of wife and mother—and thus prevent wholesale societal upheaval—they had to remove a woman's power to choose.

And so the American right-to-life movement, with the help of "pro-family" activists like Phyllis Schlafly, Christian fundamentalist preachers, and right-wing politicians, unabashedly touted the Bible-rooted construct of the "good woman" as a selfless mother above all else. They encouraged women to take their place in the "natural order" of the world—a hierarchy with god at the top, then men, then women, whose duty it was to have children. Terminating pregnancy was an assault on the very will of god. *Fetuses were people and abortionists were killing them.* The language of the debate was growing ever more heated and violent, and it was only a matter of time before actions would begin living up to the rhetoric.

In 1979, in what was said to be the first terrorist attack against an abortion clinic in the US, a firebomb destroyed Bill Baird's abortion clinic in Hempstead, Long Island. Of all the providers I'd met through NAAF, I was closest to Bill, and the news that his clinic had been bombed was incredibly upsetting. A man seen picketing the week before had walked into the clinic, screamed that everyone would burn in hell, poured gasoline across the lobby, and lit it with a torch. Thanks to Bill's careful preparation for such an attack, the only person injured had been the bomber. He was caught by the clinic's staff and sentenced to two years in a mental institution.

The case was viewed as tragic, but ultimately seen as an aberration—after all, how could "right to life" believers be capable of killing people? The claim was made that anyone who would commit such an act must be mentally ill, but time would reveal anti-abortion violence to be a serious existential threat.

I felt the severity of this war beginning to hit very close to home. In response to the escalating anti-abortion tension, I held an open house at Choices, inviting local politicians and interested parties to help me spread awareness about the city's newly declared Abortion Rights Week. I became a regular representative of the pro-choice position on radio and television programs covering abortion. As the issue became hotter, diplomatic discussions morphed into gladiatorial games, and before long I was routinely pitted against antis in heated debates.

MEANWHILE I BEGAN paying careful attention to the band of dedicated protesters who regularly picketed Choices. They were out there rain or shine. Every Saturday a priest and a group of his parishioners, mainly older women, bore signs, rosaries, and pictures of aborted fetuses to influence the young women who hurried past them into the clinic.

There was one woman in particular who hardly ever missed a Saturday. One morning I watched her as she stood just outside the clinic doors at her usual post.

She stopped a young black woman, touching her shoulder, her voice insisting, "There is another way. Choose life, let your baby live. Don't murder your own child!" The girl, shaken and frightened, pulled away and walked quickly into Choices to resolve her already difficult decision.

A man and a woman approached the doors. This time the faithful protester stood squarely in front of them, eyes blazing, fingers furiously working her rosary. "Your baby must live. How can you murder your own child?"

"Get out of my way, lady! I have a nine-year-old at home who drives me crazy. You want to take her?"

They brushed her aside. She moved on to tug at another woman's sleeve, physically trying to prevent her from entering the clinic. It was time to intervene. A Choices staff member dialed 911. A young Irish cop showed up and informed the woman that she was not to physically harass patients, that her expression of political and religious passions were limited by law.

The cop turned to the protester. "You should see them the way I have, the kids who no one wants . . . burned, scalded with boiling water, thrown out of windows."

But that reality never touched this protester or the millions like her, the people who, in turning toward the rights of fetuses, turned against the mothers who carried them.

The indefatigability of the antis has always impressed me. I cannot dismiss the passion, persistence, and power of the members of their movement. Many of the anti-choice women I have encountered over the years have been intelligent, serious activists. Many have made sacrifices to continue their activism. In light of their belief that fetuses are babies and abortionists are killing them—abortion is murder—their actions and activities are understandable. What person of conscience would not fight against the wholesale slaughter of innocents? They want to convince the world of the righteousness of their position, and they see themselves as warriors in a transcendent battle.

That is exactly how I have always felt.

On some very basic level, I understand those antis who protest outside Choices. And I respect them for acting on their beliefs—even if I will do everything in my power, and put my life on the line, to ensure that they are defeated.

IN 1980 the anti-choice movement elected one of their own to the White House to inspire, encourage, and solidify their position. With Ronald Reagan's election there was a collective joy in the air, an expression of unity and expectation among conservatives not unlike the early days of Obama's presidency. Reagan was outspokenly allied with the Moral Majority.

A year later, another Human Life amendment was introduced: the Hatch amendment, an attempt to overturn *Roe* as a federal protection and send the power to legislate abortion back to the states. With Reagan in office and a Republican majority in the Senate, the amendment posed a real threat to reproductive freedom.

I wrote a letter to Senator Hatch outlining why I was opposed. "Any federal 'human life' legislation that throws control of these issues back to the states is tantamount to a states' rights 'emancipation proclamation,' giving the states the power to decide who should be free and who should not," I wrote. "Freedom and liberty should have no boundaries. No woman should have to travel from one state to another to seek adequate medical care. . . . There is only one State—the United States—and its history and constitution cannot be prostituted."

Although the Hatch amendment did not pass, "choice," a word made dirty in the mouths of Reagan and his Moral Majority talking heads, was being attacked from all sides. As usual, the poor and those with the least access to the medical system were the first casualties. The billion dollar over-the-counter birth control industry began running misleading ads for sponges and spermicides, implying that these products were just as effective as the Pill and other prescription birth control. The companies advertised lower costs and greater ease of use without the risk of any side effects.[12] It was an egregious case of false advertising. Every day at Choices women and young girls waiting to have their abortions would earnestly insist, "But I *did* use something!" Poor women who could not access doctors as easily to receive prescription birth control were quick to buy these inexpensive sponges and spermicides. Many women were also turning to over-the-counter contraceptives because of heightened public concern about the side effects of the pill and IUDs.

I lodged complaints with members of Congress and went to work publicly accusing the drug companies of forcing women to play Russian roulette with their birth control. The *American Journal of Obstetrics and Gynecology*, *Women Wise*, and the *Los Angeles Times* published my concerns, and I had high hopes when the Food and Drug Administration finally issued a report stating that the labeling of over-the-counter products was misleading and dangerous. A bill stipulating that every over-the-counter device would have to carry labels describing how effective they were was introduced in Congress.

It didn't pass, of course; it seemed Congress wasn't keen on regulating the drug companies. Still, the defeat was baffling. Better birth control meant fewer abortions—why couldn't Republicans see that? No matter how much people disagreed about abortion, everyone should have been able to agree on the urgent need for accurate labeling and promotion of all devices that could keep women from getting pregnant against their wishes.

It was clear that with Reagan's election we had entered a new social era. Women's issues were losing popularity, while family values, American supremacy, and a unified expression of the American dream had taken center stage in public consciousness. The pro-choice movement was losing ground, and Reagan was leading the attack.

I had to find a way to fight back with something more potent than my articles and letters. In the months since my first television appearances I'd honed my natural talent for going head to head with formidable opponents. I was fascinated by the preachers on the Sunday morning shows—Jimmy Swaggart, the Church of Truth, Jerry Falwell—and I practiced debating by talking back to the television. Marty would go crazy and demand that I "turn that shit off," but I loved listening to their theatrics, especially Swaggart's. His preaching was so musical, so sensual, especially when he started speaking in tongues. I was interested in what these shows could teach me about "the enemy," but there were also points of congruence. I could relate to the preachers' overriding desire to be good, to be worthy, and I agreed with their attacks on consumerism and materialism. In fact, I even concurred with some of their diagnoses of societal problems; it was the etiology and the treatment that was at issue.

I went to see Swaggart in person once when he appeared at Madison Square Garden. A religious Jew who sat near me told me he had begun to see the light after listening to him preach. Swaggart didn't manage to "save" me, but I learned something about myself that day. I had a message as well, and it was time to begin my odyssey to spread it.

Early in 1981 I began to travel the country on a debate circuit to share my perceptions of Reagan with others who were also out in the cold. With the help of my public relations agent I arranged my own tour, traveling from the small towns in the Midwest, to the wine counties of Southern California, to industrial, forbidding Detroit, and home to Philadelphia to bring my messages regarding women, abortion, pluralism, and civil rights to any place willing to put me on the air or give me a debate. At that time I was one of the very few pro-choice activists debating the leaders of the anti-choice movement: Joe Riley, Jeanne Head, Reverend Dan Fore, Beverly LaRossa, and Kathy Quinn, among others.

I had recently conducted a two-year study at Choices in conjunction with HIP and Adelphi University, in which my patients were asked to give their reasons for having abortions. Fifty-three percent said financial reasons were the most important factor, up thirteen percentage points from a similar study done the previous year.

I called the study "Abortionomics" and publicized it widely. I wanted these findings to hit home with worshipers of Reagan, that champion of the unborn who was clearly swelling the ranks of the aborted with his economic policies. The study showed that under the influence of the Reaganomics cult, which preached and reinforced individualism, careerism, and material benefit, women were choosing mortgage payments and second cars over second babies. Women may not have seen any connection between their choice of abortion and the economic policies that led them to it, but the specter of the "Welfare Queen" planted dread in the hearts of many who might otherwise have chosen to have more children. Reagan had successfully managed to address issues of personal pain with a fluency of script that enabled people to believe that their problems were a result of misplaced "liberal values" instead of a symptom of general social and political decline.

The *New York Times* published a letter I wrote in 1984 when a seventeen-year-old student in Pennsylvania chose to have her baby and was dismissed from the National Honor Society as a consequence. Had she had an abortion, she would have been able to remain in the society. "What a set of circumstances in a country which gives lip service to the concept that it is a good thing for women to have children, yet punishes some of them so severely when they choose to do so," I wrote. "The time is long past for women to stop being victimized by a society whose double messages place them in the position of always being wrong. One wonders, too, about the male involved in this pregnancy. Will he be allowed his 'honors'?"

My study also revealed a powerful contradiction: the majority of women who came to the clinic for the purpose of having an abortion did not consider themselves to be pro-choice. They had never imagined themselves in a position where they would decide to have an abortion, an act they considered morally reprehensible even as they waited their turns to be called into the operating rooms. Many shunned the pro-choice movement and distanced themselves from other women who had gone through the same thing. Colleagues told me of women who picketed their clinics, came inside for abortions, then went right back to the picket lines.

As long as women judged themselves by Reagan's vision of a "good mother," they would also judge one another. It was a defense mechanism, a way to protect themselves against the shame and guilt they had internalized. In a heightened state of self-preservation they created a wall between individual experience and collective understanding. Many politely shook their heads when I asked them to sign petitions, come to rallies, or participate in meetings. Some women, faced with the challenge of being harassed on their way into the clinic, became briefly politicized as a way to express their anger, but few actively joined the pro-choice movement. After their abortions, most women just wanted to leave it all behind.

Yet despite this desire for distance, women demonstrated a quiet solidarity with the cause through the simple act of having them. They referred their friends and family to Choices for abortions and came back to the clinic every time they needed counseling or care. Women were silently, undeniably connected to each other by the necessity of making reproductive choices. Every woman who chose abortion took part in an ongoing struggle toward a "reluctant epiphany," a realization that not politics, but necessity drives women's choices—and thus, there is an inherent morality in having the power to choose.

There were some women who did have the courage to vocalize their experiences and take action, however small. I remember one woman in particular who I met on my debate tour that year. She had been a prostitute on welfare, using sex to get by after her second marriage. She said she was forty, but she looked much older. As we walked through the quiet campus where I was scheduled to speak that day, she told me that her abortions had been an expected occupational hazard. Now she sat on several boards of directors, a pillar of her community. Listening to her, I felt a sense of awe and wonder. So many activists are made, not born, radicalized by life, not theory.

On a trip to Todos Santos, California, I was to be the keynote speaker at a professional women's conference. These women were hungry for inspiration. They came to their activism the hard way, not on college campuses or in consciousness-raising groups, but through marriages. Most of them were divorced. When I finished my talk, a woman got up and began, "I've never told anyone about it, but five years ago I got pregnant and I had an abortion . . ." With that, she had joined the movement. She'd found her voice and reached out to her sisters.

That was what I lived for, the small awakenings and profound beginnings. And I finally had enough psychological distance to recognize the phenomenon and call myself a feminist.

I RETURNED TO NEW YORK that summer for a nationally televised debate with a prominent anti-choice leader. I was anxious and tremendously concerned that I should win.

I understood that one could never really convert the other side. Debates merely served to rearticulate the issues on an ever higher and more conscious level so that those already converted became disciples.

My debate was taped on a Friday. I had taken a pregnancy test that morning, leaving my urine at Choices. My period was a couple of weeks late, and I was worried. I was always so careful, almost obsessive, but no method of birth control is perfect.

As the debate progressed, I experienced an odd sort of splitting off. I responded to the gibes and questions of my opponent, all the while thinking that I could be pregnant. I felt removed enough to appreciate the irony of the situation, a battle being waged on multiple tracks. I was performing politically for the cameras and debating emotionally with myself. My opponent asked me how I could call myself a feminist and support abortion rights when half the fetuses being aborted were female. It was not a new argument. None of it was, but this time it made me think of my mother. My mother, with dreams deferred and denied.

In the closing argument I made a passionate plea for the importance of women's lives, for remembering that the abortion "issue" was ultimately about that. Thousands of individual stories, thousands of different reasons, all culminating in one shared ambiguous reality—a reality I was beginning to enter.

I finished the taping and asked to use the studio phone to call my office. The assistant stood next to me, engaging me in conversation; I was talking, laughing. Then I got on the phone, spoke to my secretary, and found out that the pregnancy test was positive. It took my breath away.

Sweating profusely, I wondered whether I had stained the outfit I was wearing for the debate. I called a cab, flattened my back against the seat, and took slow, deep breaths, trying to keep from feeling suffocated. The idea of abortion was a valve, an opening, a way to breathe. There was no question of whether I would have one. As we crossed the Fifty-Ninth Street Bridge, I held my stomach and said aloud, "Sorry little one, it's just not time."

My diary entry from that night reads, "For one night I am a mother." I don't remember whether or not I slept. I only remember my exhaustion and an overriding sense of inevitability. The next morning I dressed carefully in a red-and-white suit. What does one wear to an abortion? There are no traditional costumes like those for funerals or weddings. There is no ritual from one generation of women to another to look to as a guide. There are only functional considerations; you wear something that comes on and off quickly and easily.

At Choices, the steps of the familiar process played out in surreal reversal. The blood tests, the images of the sonogram, the table, the stirrups—they were all for me. Marty stood at the head of the table and held my hand while Dr. Mohammed performed the abortion. Now I was joined to the common experience of my sex. But as I lay on the table I had stood beside to support so many others, I felt irrevocably alone. The hands that touched and caressed my hair felt as if they moved through a dark porous divide that separated me from everything that I knew or had been before. As I spread my legs like all my sisters, I thought of the child whose time was not now. Strange how I thought of the fetus as female, as if that shared gender gave me a more special connection.

Yet despite that connection—the recognition of the fetus's potential to become my child—I knew that I could not allow this pregnancy to come to term. My sense of self, my sense of time, the flow of my movement toward goals that I had created had been interrupted the moment my test came back positive. The fetus was an invader, a separate force growing inside me, demanding and creating potentially unalterable realities. I couldn't let my life become someone else's.

St. Thomas Aquinas wrote that each individual operates by the "law of self-preservation," the instinctive tendency we have to survive at all costs. The Catholic Church's just war doctrine accepts the taking of human life if one's life or that of another is directly threatened, in keeping with Aquinas's "natural law."[13] Does the fetus not impede a woman's tendency to maintain her own existence? Is it not an unjust aggressor, threatening the survival of the mother? Is not a woman's choice of abortion an act of self-defense? With my choice I was fighting for the right of all women to define abortion as an act of love: love for the family one already has, and just as important, love for oneself. I was fighting to reclaim abortion as a mother's act. It was an act of solidarity as significant as any other I had committed.

After my abortion, as I slowly awoke from the anesthesia, I became conscious of immense and overwhelming feelings: non-specific, non-directed. Love, relief—then sadness.

A few days later, walking down the hallway in Choices, I heard loud, wrenching sobs coming from the recovery room. A woman was waking from anesthesia and crying for her mother. I went to her bed, lowered the side rails, and gently tried to soothe her. As I bent down to her face she whispered in a halting Russian accent, "You're the only one I have now, I'm all alone. You've saved my life by being here." I held the woman close, enormously moved, savoring our connection. There was no good or bad, no issue of choice. There was nothing more than the pure energy of survival, and women doing what they had been doing for centuries throughout history, what they will do forever.

MARTY AND I didn't talk much about my abortion. He was never one to feel comfortable articulating his feelings, but I know he must have had a deep reaction. Oh, how silence can palpate, how distance between self and other can be stretched, distorted, choked with expectations not met. I had learned very early on how to deal with invisibility in my relationship with my father. Marty's silence left me in the same place.

Years later he told me that if I had become pregnant during our affair, he would have immediately left his wife to marry me. I was shocked when I heard that. Although I knew that pregnancy was often used as a tool in relationships, it never occurred to me to use it in ours.

The distance between Marty and me after the abortion had become characteristic of our relationship. In our early days together there had been no question of who was the teacher and who was the pupil. But now I'd passed him by on multiple levels, and my progress became one more obstacle to intimacy between us. Our competition with each other was like a blood sport, and our relationship thinned a little each time a cut was made. He was still proud of me, but the pride was mixed with envy of my youth, my public prominence, and my future. Once, when we were lying in bed together, he turned to me with that loving look, now shaded with sadness, and asked whether we could declare a cease-fire. I gently touched his cheek, whispering my assent.

After the crescendo of our wedding, we had fallen into a comfortably numbing routine. Garrison had become a kind of beautiful green prison. We would eat dinner together and then go to our corners, his in the den, where he smoked his pipe, and mine in the bedroom where I retreated to read. Or I'd take solitary walks on the Appalachian Trail while Marty puttered about or watched a game. I hated the sounds of those games. I remembered them coming from my father's den, the constant screams of the crowd over some ball.

And then there were the politics of sleep. Marty always said that bed was only for sleeping or fucking, but for me it was a womb, a final port of safety, a place where I could be most free, both in body and mind. I loved to take to my bed to read, write, talk on the phone for hours with friends, letting sleep come naturally when it may. But no matter the stress of the day or the passion of the night, Marty went to bed at exactly eleven thirty, right after the news. I couldn't talk with him, read, or even move for fear of disturbing him. Eventually, I had to move out of our bedroom.

When we traveled, our marriage felt like a continuation of the excitement of our affair. Abroad, we could be ourselves, with no expectations from others. We went on cruises to Alaska, safaris in Africa, visited beautiful hidden spas in the winter wonderlands of Scandinavia. Marty took me back to the Carlton Hotel in France, and this time we shared a suite overlooking the Mediterranean with my little dog Noodles. I sunned on the beach at Cannes without a bra, feeling totally comfortable with Marty by my side. He loved to show me off, and I reveled in his admiration. And yet, I remember watching the students lazily camped out on the beach in Cannes as I walked along the tree-lined avenues, wishing myself with them, envying their freedom. I had the feeling that my marriage was a garment that never quite fit. I was always attempting to move quickly, to stretch, to turn, to run, and even sometimes to dance—a Dionysian dance, one of release and forgetting—but that was impossible.

I tried to find ways to bridge the distance between us. Once, I came home on a Saturday to Garrison from a particularly intense meeting at Brooklyn Law School where Shere Hite had spoken. I was filled with philosophy and the danger of the ideas we had discussed. It was summer, and Marty was in the kitchen preparing dinner. I wanted to talk to him about the meeting, but he could not engage on any level except a sarcastic one. He wouldn't even turn off the faucet so he could hear what I had to say. I gave up and went outside to set the table, my head spinning from the tension of my competing realities.

Guests we invited offered a bit of relief from what I often experienced as a deadening sameness. One evening Barry Feinstein, one of New York's most politically influential labor leaders (who was later revealed to have embezzled union funds), came to our house for dinner. My experience as president of NAAF and the success of my debate tour had led me to consider entering electoral politics, and I asked him his opinion on whether I should throw my hat in the proverbial ring. "Who the hell do you think you are?" he answered. "How do you think you could do anything in politics? You are a woman from Westchester who gives great parties."

Another time Harold Fisher, then the chairman of the Metropolitan Transit Authority (MTA), floated in my indoor pool in his black glasses, pontificating on the nature of realpolitik. I sat at the pool's edge and argued my stance on an abortion bill that had been brought to the state senate. When I asked for his help and support, he dismissively replied, "There are no issues—only elections."

I turned to animals to ease some of the loneliness and boredom I felt at home. I would respond to pleas on the radio from the local shelters: "If someone calls in the next two hours, you can save this cat's or dog's life." Many of my companion animals came into my life that way.

On one of my long walks I became friendly with a neighbor who lived at the bottom of the mountain. She had a riding stable and led horse and pony treks on the Appalachian

Trail. I began going for rides with her as often as possible, but I soon grew tired of having to live by my neighbor's schedule. It wasn't long before I felt the desire to create my own equestrian world. I cleared two acres of rocky, mountainous land, built an eight-stall barn, and filled it with horses.

The barn became my private space. I approached riding with the same discipline that had kept me at the piano playing obsessively, and I would practice the delicate, difficult moves of dressage in the indoor ring for hours. I rode alone on the paths behind my land, writing speeches in my head. I loved jumping most of all; there is something extraordinary about flying on a two-thousand-pound animal—the degree of trust it involves, the courage of both horse and rider, the complete fusion of two bodies and minds at that one moment of suspension. With my horses there was no need for translation, no fear of misunderstandings. Our communication was clear and direct, with no detours through ego.

I WAS ALWAYS CAPABLE of hiding my inner turmoil from professional colleagues and political allies, conscious of projecting an image of impenetrable grace and power. I had become a feminist in solitude, separated from the movement and the writers of my time. This had its benefits: my perceptions were less contaminated by theory or polemics. But I was ready to strengthen my connection to other feminists, to join and help direct the feminist movement. Almost in defiance of the hermetic lifestyle I led with Marty and his difficulty in communicating with me intellectually, I decided to embark on a new project that would place me at the center of the network of feminists who I perceived were shaping the politics of the times.

We were still in the early years of legalization, and despite Reagan's war on abortion, feminists had enough sway to influence the way the issue was handled in the media and reach out to those who'd been victimized by the guilt and judgment that characterized those years. After years of writing pamphlets, educational materials, and newspaper articles, I felt that the most effective way to communicate my personal and political ideas and catalyze a network of others who shared my values would be through a print publication that could be distributed to patients and mailed to pro-choice constituents and fellow feminists.

I started by publishing an eight-page Choices newsletter. I opened the first issue with the Euripides quotation "Woman is woman's natural ally" and wrote of my experience founding Choices and the catalytic inspiration of my patients. I purchased large mailing lists of health providers, women's groups, student health centers—any organization I thought would be interested—and sent out thirty thousand free copies of the newsletter.

It wasn't long before letters began pouring in. People wrote to me about the topics we covered, thanked me for publishing the newsletter, and even sent checks with their requests for more issues. Carolyn Handel, a cousin of mine who had worked in advertising and sales with the magazine *High Times,* suggested I take advantage of the groundswell and publish a real magazine with subscriptions and advertising. Not knowing anything about publishing, I did what came naturally: I jumped in headfirst and learned as I went. Carolyn started selling ads and promoting the vision, I recruited more writers, we published quarterly, and before I knew it, *On the Issues* magazine was alive and growing.

Subsequent editions covered the symbols and rallies of the pro-choice movement, the fundamental tenets of Patient Power, and the important work of pro-choice organizations like NAF. Feminist projects, workshops, and meetings were announced and promoted in every issue. No topic was off limits: I included articles on obstacles faced by women of color, systemic inequalities that affected gays and lesbians, international women's rights, and animal rights. Articles were contributed by pro-choice activists, prominent feminists, providers, doctors, and even patients who had a message they wanted to share. The magazine gave me a long-sought-after intellectual peer group. It stimulated my thinking, functioned as an educational tool, and provided a forum for philosophical discussions. It was exactly what I needed.

Exhilarated by the success of *On the Issues,* wanting my ideas to reach even more people, I wrote, co-produced, and directed a thirty-minute film titled *Abortion: A Different Light,* which aired on several cable channels and reached eleven million homes. I structured the film as a group of interviews, a collection of stories related to abortion. Pro-choice leaders and Choices staff told moving stories of their experiences with the issue. Marty described his experiences on the "Midnight Express" and spoke about the struggles doctors faced in helping women who were hospitalized for attempting self-abortions, and Bill Baird described the fire-bombing of his clinic. I included a few clips from my debates and interviewed Lawrence Lader, longtime abortion rights advocate, Sarah Weddington, the lawyer for the plaintiff in *Roe,* and others.

The stories these providers and politicians told were illuminating, but I thought the true beauty of my film lay in the interviews with patients about their personal experiences. Their voices served as a form of resistance to the public's obsessive focus on the fetus, a way to recenter the issue of reproductive rights in the reality of women's lives, where it belonged.

The most striking of these voices was that of one of my

first patients, Helen Cole, a Catholic who had been against abortion until that moment came when she knew she had to have one. When I approached her to ask if she would participate in the film, she told me it would be very difficult for her to talk about her abortion. Then she met my gaze. "I want to be in your film," she said. "It will be my gift to you and the movement." The memory of her courage and generosity will always be with me.

IN 1982, I spoke to a large audience at a NOW meeting in Rockland County:

> Tonight when I use the words "anti-abortion" I want you to put in their place "anti-women." For whoever would drive women to butchers again, whoever would deprive them of freedom and liberty in the name of god, law, or politics—is most surely their enemy. We must never forget that beyond the words, the fanaticism, the debates, the discussions, there are grown women who must not be sacrificed on the altars of unanswered and unanswerable questions of when life begins and who and when and if it should be protected. We must never allow women to be manipulated and pressured by political struggles between the church and state or fall victims of a religious holy war. For underlying all opposition to abortion, all attempts at restrictive legislation, is a vocal and virulent minority who are attempting to impose their own personal belief of the immorality of abortion on all of us.
>
> . . . There is only one absolute truth in regard to abortion and that is that it must remain a matter of personal decision and private conscience. Liberty and freedom to choose, like breathing, eating, walking, and loving, are rights granted to us by a higher authority than Senators Hatch, Helms, or Hyde!

In the ten years since the creation of Flushing Women's, the clinic had gone from serving five patients per week to becoming a nationally recognized model of a successful women's health care facility. I decided to throw a "Revolutionary Ball," a costume party to celebrate Choices' tenth anniversary. It would be held at the St. Regis Hotel, and I would invite all the political players who had been involved from the start. Everyone was required to dress as their revolutionary hero.

The event was covered in Page Six of the *Post*, with the humorous headline, "Labor Big Shots Frolic In Fancy Costumes." The great fun of having a political costume ball allowed otherwise serious heavyweights to play. Marty went as George Washington, in silk hose and a ruffled shirt. President of the Sanitation Union Ed Ostrowski was Thomas Jefferson, Jack Bigel was Lafayette, and Harold Fisher, the ex-MTA chief, came as Henry George, the nineteenth-century economist who pushed for a onetime land tax. Others came costumed as George Sand, Madame Roland, and Martha Washington. I was Fanny Wright, with a high white wig and a wide crinoline gown.

That night, I was completely in my element. So much had happened in the last decade. I'd helped pioneer and define an entirely new world. Traveling the country, debating on television, delivering my message to crowds of women, I was more myself than I had ever been. I felt a sense of completeness, happiness in the knowledge that my entire being was in use, as if every part of me was active and interactive. The light of the passion for my work kept the struggles of my marriage in the shadows.

The Politics of Courage

*"A life beset with danger is always
the best school for acquiring a brave spirit."*
—JOHANNES MÜLLER,
HINDRANCES OF LIFE (1909)

Miss Hoffman," he said, "how many abortions did your facility do last year?" I was debating Jerry Falwell in Detroit in 1983 on national television.

"Reverend, I believe we did nine thousand abortions," I told him proudly. To my thinking this high number was a measure of the excellence of our work. Like any medical practice, any business, the more people who come to you, the better your services are assumed to be.

But to Falwell's ears it was a measure of mass murder.

"When you meet your maker with the blood of nine thousand babies on your hands, what will you say? How will you justify that?"

"Reverend, when I meet *her*, I will be very proud, because I fought and struggled for women's rights."

"Her? Her? Are you saying god is a woman?"

"No, Reverend," I said. "God is beyond gender."

A woman in the audience rose, obviously distraught, her voice shaking. She relayed her own experience with abortion:

the guilt still with her, the doctor's coldness, how "they"—the abortion doctors—would not let her see her child. She extended her hand, pointed an accusing finger at me, and declared, "You are nothing but a Hitler to me."

Her words shot out at me like bullets. It was useless to attempt to respond to this angry woman. Caught in the same battle all women were fighting, drowning in her own society-inflicted guilt, she was only repeating the popular anti-choice rhetoric of the day.

By the mid-eighties we were firmly in the midst of a backlash against the calls for equality of the seventies. Women struggled to find their place among men who had not accepted the ideas put forward by feminism, entering the workforce in droves while deflecting the cry for "family values" that screamed at them from newspapers, the streets, inside their homes.

Men raged at women for having reneged on the traditional expectation that their primary role should be that of nurturer and total support system. They raged against women's expressions of sexuality, their recently acquired right to choose, and the continuing and escalating feminist demands for power and participation in society. Most of all, they raged against the radical new world order that female power represented.

This rage reared its head in casual conversations and was present in images of women in the media. It was as ubiquitous in the workplace as it was in the home. Often, it took the form of physical violence. Humiliations faced us each morning as we scanned the media reports. A 1987 *New York Times* article reported that there were six million battered women in the United States that year;[14] experts estimated that a woman was battered every fifteen seconds. The constant threat of violence served to reinforce and institutionalize men's physical and societal dominance over women.

Of course legal abortion, a symbol of the penultimate right of women to have power over their bodies and reproductive lives, became the natural public focus of this backlash against feminism. As Susan Faludi wrote, it was a "counterassault on women's rights . . . an attempt to retract the handful of small and hard-won victories the feminist movement did manage to win for women."[15] Deeply frustrated by their inability to get Human Life legislation passed, fundamentalist zealots bent on removing this civil right decided to take matters into their own hands.

Their aggression toward abortion clinics and providers first manifested through increasingly violent language. The word "choice" was positioned against "life," diminishing the one and empowering the other so that "pro-choice" came to mean pro-death, pro-murder. As the angry rhetoric of the anti-choice movement intensified, I noticed a growing tendency to liken abortion to the Holocaust, to compare the private moral decisions of individual women to the wholesale slaughter of Jews during the Second World War. An abortion clinic in Westchester was labeled "Auschwitz on the Hudson," and anti-abortion protesters raised placards with Nazi insignias in front of clinics across the country. Pseudoscientific books were written detailing Nazi experiments in concentration camps and their supposed similarities to procedures in abortion clinics, and the specter of Hitler's death camps abounded in terminology like "Abortoriums" and "Child Killing Centers." This analogy between Jews and fetuses was an effective way to humanize fetuses, casting them as victims deserving of civil rights.

Comparisons between fetuses and black slaves achieved the same end. The first time I heard the Civil War analogy used to describe the abortion struggle was in 1983 when I debated Nellie Gray, an anti-abortion leader who coordinated the annual January 22 March for Life on Washington. An early attempt at finding "common ground" failed miserably when I suggested we work together to reduce the need for abortion by educating women on birth control and making it more available. During a break in our taping, she said, "You know, this is just like the Lincoln-Douglas debates on slavery." I smiled in recognition until I realized that she was positioning me as Douglas. "We'll stop our attacks and talk about birth control when you put down your knives and stop the killing," she told me.

Pro-lifers played fast and loose with demonizing metaphors, and put themselves on the side of angels when it suited their strategic purposes. Even as they compared the atrocities of the Holocaust to abortion, they accused Jews and lesbians of running the abortion industry for "blood money." They publicly equated abortion with the United States' history of slavery, but told African American patients outside of Choices that they were desecrating the legacy of Dr. Martin Luther King. They stopped at nothing.

The incendiary atmosphere the leaders of the anti-choice movement created around the abortion issue was fuel for religious fervor among their followers. Cardinal John J. O'Connor, the archbishop of New York and a leading voice in the anti-abortion movement, riled his disciples with Mother Teresa's assertion that "the greatest enemy to world peace is abortion." Reproductive freedom and women's lives were now not merely synonymous with murder, but a threat to world peace. If fetuses were being murdered, then the women choosing abortion were committing genocide against their own race. Every woman became a murderess, or potential one.

Women trying to exert control over their own bodies were working in league with the devil against the sacred Christian hierarchy. One speaker famously stated at an anti-choice rally, "Ask my son who's boss and he'll say Mommy. Ask my wife who's boss and she'll tell you it's me. My wife submits to me because I submit to god." Antis projected their fears of powerlessness and social disorder onto the fetus, becoming its "saviors." And of course, a savior stops at nothing when it comes to eliminating the enemy.

But for whom, exactly, were they fighting? Few but the most religiously fanatical would wage a hot war in the name of a group of cells. No, this war was being fought *against* women, not *for* fetuses, and they had found an ingenious way of disguising that truth: they began calling it a baby and emphasizing the developments that made it recognizable as human. At eight weeks the fetus's heartbeat could be detected; at twelve, it could bend its thumb; at fourteen, it could breathe amniotic fluid.

Photos of fetuses, however, didn't make for effective propaganda; they weren't cute enough, human enough. Because humans seem to be hardwired to respond to animals that have certain facial characteristics—big eyes, round heads, and short snouts—antis began comparing fetuses to helpless animals. Nat Hentoff, writing in the *Village Voice*, asked his readers to imagine the fetus as a baby seal, assuming that all the protective feelings one would naturally get while viewing an adorable white pup being clubbed to death could be transferred to a fetus floating in its mother's womb.

This drive to encourage a reflexive empathy with the fetus was expressed perfectly at a right-to-life conference I attended with Bill Baird, where an Australian priest described to a hushed audience the ten-day fast he had conducted in a public square to "get in touch with the helplessness and defenselessness of the fetus." A slide show began. It showed a funeral, a small casket, hundreds of marchers each carrying one rose, tears, speeches, an interment. "Mary Elizabeth," a four-month fetus supposedly rescued from a garbage can and posthumously named and celebrated, appeared on the screen with the caption, "Victim of the abortion holocaust." Moving through the crowd, I saw fetuses floating in bottles of formaldehyde. Everyone seemed to be wearing mother-of-pearl pins on their lapels. Looking closer, I saw it was their logo: tiny fetal feet, on sale for three dollars.

The concept of the fetus as independent from the mother reached its apotheosis in Bernard Nathanson's 1984 film *Silent Scream*, which supposedly showed a fetus withdrawing in fear during a second trimester abortion procedure. The patient, however, was absent; the film never showed anything but the fetus in utero, its mother's womb looking like some subterranean ecosystem. You might have thought the woman didn't exist at all.

Unable to make their choices in a vacuum, women were forced to endure the psychological, and often physical, trauma of entering a public war with the antis and a private war with their own bodies. The more symbolic and legal independence the fetus gained, the less agency women had over their own reproductive choices.

Human Life Amendments, while never passed, were still frequently brought to the table, and judicial concern for fetal welfare and rights began to escalate. Court cases addressing policies in which employers selectively barred pregnant women—or even women who were not pregnant, but of childbearing age—from specific jobs because of a "threat to the fetus" became increasingly common. In a ruling for one company, the court stated that "an unborn child's exposure to lead creates a substantial health risk involving the danger of permanent harm."

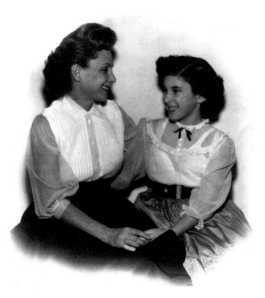

My mother Ruth and me,
Philadelphia, 1955.

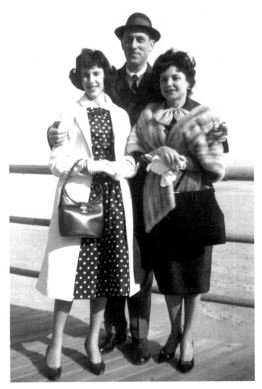

My father Jack holds both of
us close on the boardwalk in
Atlantic City, 1959.

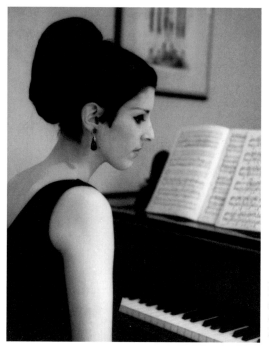

At home in Queens,
New York, preparing
for a recital at
Chatham Square
Music School, 1964.

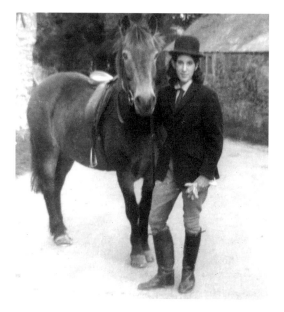

Ready for the hunt,
Cornwall, England,
1968.

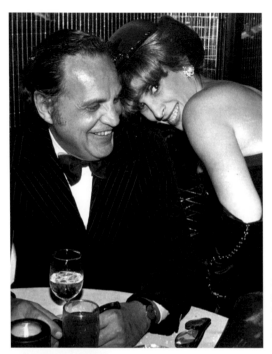

Marty and me at a glamorous fundraising dinner for breast cancer programs, New York City, circa 1980s.

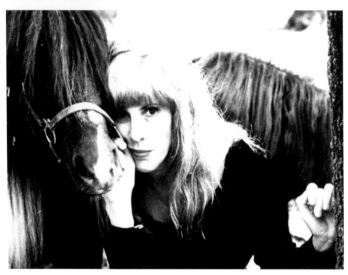

With my horses in Garrison, New York, circa 1990. PHOTO: SUZZANE FIOL.

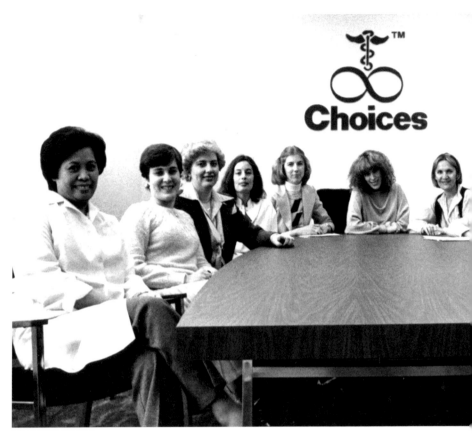

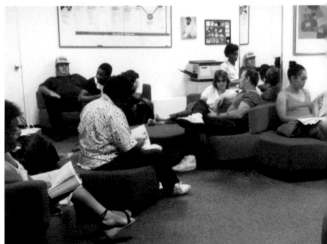

Above: My management staff in the boardroom at Choices, Queens, New York, 1980.

Right: The red and purple chairs in the waiting room at Choices, 1980.

Far right: The first issue of *On the Issues,* Fall 1983, shows the Choices connection between receptionist and patient.

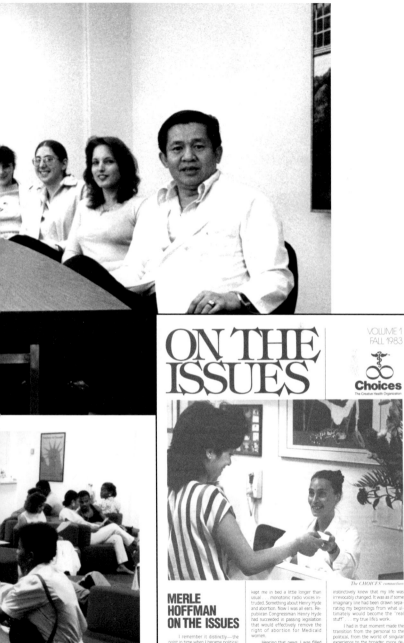

ON THE
ISSUES

VOLUME 1
FALL 1983

Choices
The Creative Health Organization

The CHOICES' connection

MERLE HOFFMAN ON THE ISSUES

I remember it distinctly—the point in time when I became political: it was summer, 1976, and the smells and sounds of a country morning kept me in bed a little longer than usual . . . monotonic radio voices intruded. Something about Henry Hyde and abortion. Now I was all ears. Republican Congressman Henry Hyde had succeeded in passing legislation that would effectively remove the right of abortion for Medicaid women.

Hearing that news, I was filled with an intense self-awareness, coupled with a strong feeling of fate. I instinctively knew that my life was irrevocably changed. It was as if some imaginary line had been drawn separating my beginnings from what ultimately would become the "real stuff" . . . my true life's work.

I had in that moment made the transition from the personal to the political, from the world of singular experience to the broader, more demanding and dangerous one of social and political activism.

continued on pg. 2

1

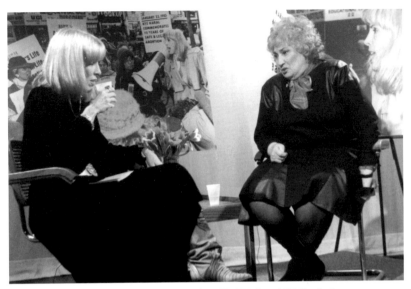

Interviewing Bella Abzug, my first guest on the cable TV show *MH: On the Issues*, New York City, 1986.

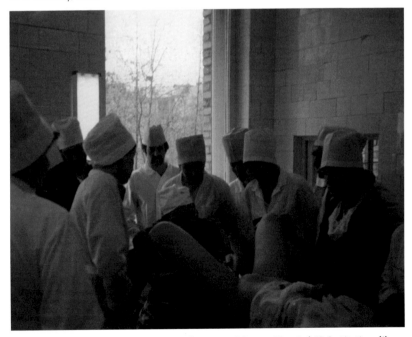

Dr. David Gluck teaching our abortion techniques at Moscow Hospital 53. Institutions like this one inspired me to fight for Russian women's reproductive rights. Moscow, Russia, 1998.

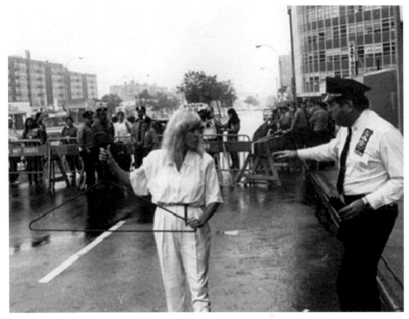

Just another Saturday morning at Choices, Queens, New York, circa 1990s.

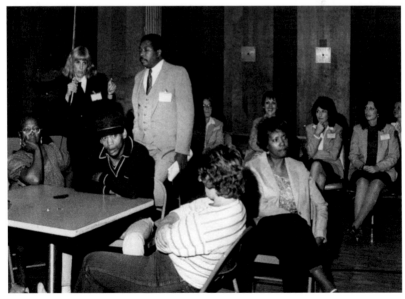

With the help of the Choices staff and the Creedmoor Mental Health Players, I am leading a workshop for inmates at Rikers Island on transitioning to the outside world, Queens, New York, circa late 1980s.

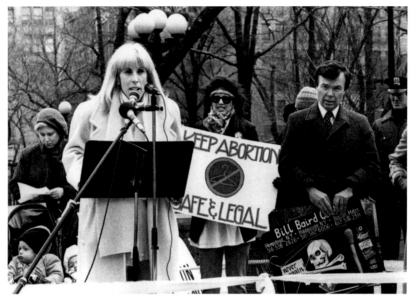

At a pro-choice rally in Union Square celebrating January 22nd, with Grace Paley (far left) and Bill Baird (far right), New York City, circa 1980s.

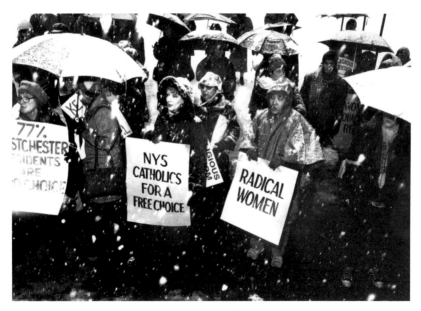

Pro-choice supporters rally in Bryant Park during a blizzard, New York City, circa 1987.

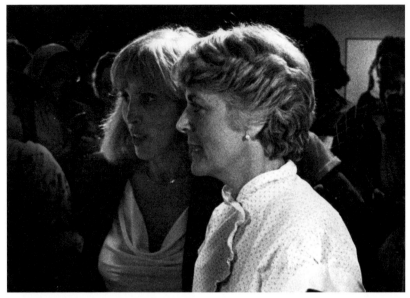

With Geraldine Ferraro, after her announcement as the Democratic vice-presidential candidate, New York City, 1984.

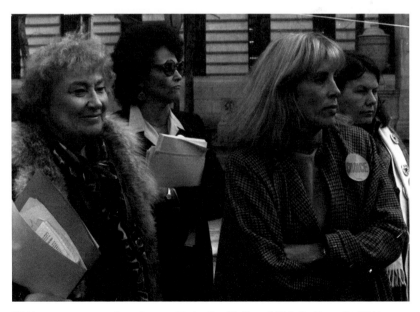

Waiting our turn to speak at a January 22nd rally with (from left) Bella Abzug, Dr. Vickie Alexander, and Betty Maloney, Bryant Park, New York City, circa 1980s.

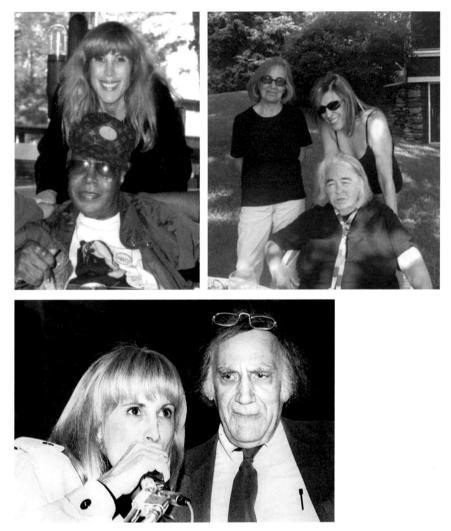

Top left: With Florynce Kennedy at an *On the Issues* retreat in my home, Garrison, New York, circa 1990.

Top right: With Mahin Hassibi (left) and Kate Millett at Kate's farm in Poughkeepsie, New York, 2008. PHOTO: MYRA KORVARY.

Bottom: On the soapbox with William Kunstler protectively at my side, at the pro-choice rally and march down Thirty-Fourth Street, New York City, 1985.

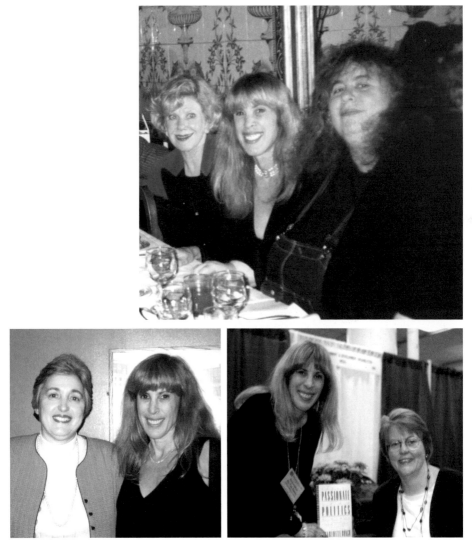

Top: With Erica Jong (left) and Andrea Dworkin at an *On the Issues* holiday party, New York City, circa 1990s.

Bottom left: With Ellie Smeal at NCAP event, circa 1990s.

Bottom right: With Charlotte Bunch at NOW conference, circa 1990s.

TAYLOR: AMEX vs. EDMOND SAFRA • WHERE TO GET A SUPER WORKOUT

$1.95 • SEPTEMBER 18, 1989

NEW YORK

ABORTION

IN NEW YORK

"When I woke up from the anesthesia, I was kind of dizzy, like [I] was in another world, and the first thing out of my mouth was 'M[y] baby.' I remember I said that and I was crying."

Ana is a sixteen-year-old high-school student from Queens. T[his] year, she has had two abortions. "The first time I got pregnant[...]

BY JEANIE KASINDORF (continued on page 32)

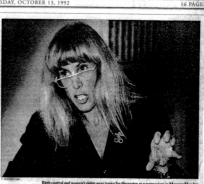

Pro-choice
demonstration in front
of St. Patrick's
Cathedral last April, and
supporter a pro-choice
protest above.

The ✠ Moscow Times

SINCE 1992

NO. 68   TUESDAY, OCTOBER 13, 1992   16 PAGES

PRO-CHOICE
COMES TO MOSCOW

By Nanette van der Laan
THE MOSCOW TIMES

Russian coast guards boarded the Greenpeace ship Solo off the islands of Novaya Zemlya Monday, detaining the entire crew for illegally trespassing in Russian territorial waters.

Coast guard personnel fired three shots across the stern of the Solo early Monday morning, according to a spokesperson for Greenpeace. The ship, with a crew of 34, is on a mission to investigate nuclear contamination in the area.

"Three shots from a 30 millimeter canon were fired at the Solo in the morning and in the afternoon two officers and 10 coast guards boarded the ship," said Eleanor O'Hanlon, the Moscow representative of Greenpeace on Monday. "We expect the ship will be escorted, on guard, to a port near Arkhangelsk."

O'Hanlon said Monday night that radio contact had been lost with the Solo. She also said that Russian officials and the environmentalists were still disputing where, precisely, the bor-

der between national and international waters lies.

The conflict began on Saturday, when the Solo was warned against crossing the Kara Straits into Russian waters and a coast-guard vessel, the Ural, set off in hot pursuit.

On Sunday the Ural shot three flares at the Greenpeace ship, which Solo's captain Albert Kuiken chose to ignore. Kuiken told O'Hanlon that although the Ural captain was threatening to use gunfire, he did not change course. He said he was sure he was not breaking any laws and was sailing in international waters, where he enjoyed the right of free passage.

By Monday morning the Solo was still in the Straits and sent a large inflatable dinghy with a crew of six to try to reach the site of a nuclear attack submarine dumped in shallow waters in 1982, according to O'Hanlon. For 40 minutes the Ural threatened to open fire while another coastguard vessel began pursuing the dinghy, Greenpeace said.

See SHIP, Page 2

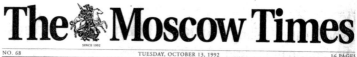

Pro-Choice   Birth control and women's rights were topics for discussion at a symposium in Moscow Monday. "Women in Russia must start taking control of their health care," said Merle Hoffman, above, a pro-choice activist and president of Choices Women's Medical Center. Page 3.

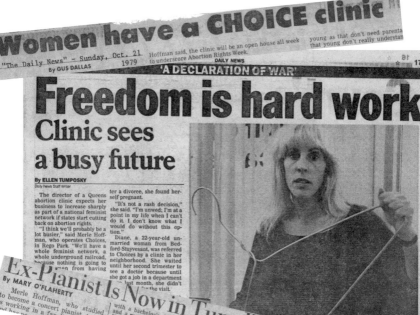

Women have a CHOICE clinic

"The Daily News" – Sunday, Oct. 21, 1979

By GUS DALLAS

Hoffman said, the clinic will be an open house all week to underscore Abortion Rights Week.

young as that don't need parental that young don't really understand

DAILY NEWS 17

'A DECLARATION OF WAR'

Freedom is hard work

Clinic sees a busy future

By ELLEN TUMPOSKY
Daily News Staff Writer

The director of a Queens abortion clinic expects her business to increase sharply as part of a national feminist network if states start cutting back on abortion rights.

"I think we'll probably be a lot busier," said Merle Hoffman, who operates Choices, in Rego Park. "We'll have a whole feminist network, a whole underground railroad, because nothing is going to keep them from having

ter a divorce, she found herself pregnant.

"It's not a rash decision," she said. "I'm unwed, I'm at a point in my life when I can't do it. I don't know what I would do without this option."

Diane, a 22-year-old unmarried woman from Bedford-Stuyvesant, was referred to Choices by a clinic in her neighborhood. She waited until her second trimester to see a doctor because until she got a job in a department ... last month, she didn't ... the visit.

with a bachelor's degree in psychology and a member of Phi Beta Kappa, Ms. Hoffman describes herself as a "social psychologist." She is now studying part time in a combined masters-doctorate program ... [City University's] abortion," she said.

She was influenced, she said, by seeing her best friend's troubled life since having a baby at age 16.

Ms. Hoffman, 31 and single, is attractive with long hair in windblown style. It's a light reddish auburn, but she says frankly, "I change the color according to my moods."

Asked ... just taking over the male roles in society without questioning the values."

Ms. Hoffman, 31 and single ... phia, came to Kew ... was 12 and now liv ...

CLINIC DIRECTOR Merle Hoffman

Ex-Pianist Is Now in Tune With Women's Health

By MARY O'FLAHERTY

Merle Hoffman, who studied to become a concert pianist, today is working in a far different field and has no ... ... the effects of ... preme Court decision ... she calls "a declaration of war" on women.

Rainbow of women

Choices, founded in 1971, sees 30,000 patients a year, half of them for abortions. Its cheerful waiting room is crowded with about 50 women — a rainbow in age, race ...

Groups Gearing Up To Do Battle in NY

RIGHTS from Page 4

tion advice center for women in Manhattan. "Now they'll have to come ou ...

ABORTION: THE HISTORIC DECISION

Angry debate still rages on D.C. sidewalk

WASHINGTON from Page 5

bia, Md., said she was disappointed the court had not banned abortion altogether.

"But it's a step in the right direction," she said.

"We just have to be patient and wait. Things have to move slow."

The crowds had gathered every day for three weeks, waiting for the court to hand down its historic ruling.

Some who were determined to hear the justices announce their opinions yesterday had lined up the night before.

Also during the night, in Concord, N.H., a deliberately set fire caused minor damage to an abortion clinic.

In Washington, soon after the bright dawn, the news that the New Hampshire clinic was the latest to be attacked raised tensions among the demonstrators.

of decision brought a brief silence to the marble plaza.

The competitive chanting ceased as attorneys and journalists feverishly turned the pages of the court's decision.

A bearded man wearing the brown robe of a Catholic friar knelt on the sidewalk, fingering the beads of a long rosary. The sign above his head stated: "The baby had no choice."

"I'm not clear what happened exactly," mused a young woman in purple shorts.

"I'm trying to figure this out."

"What does it mean?" asked another.

"It means if you've got money you can get an abortion," said Molly Yard, president of the National Organization for Women.

"If you're poor, too bad — you're down the drain."

A PUBLIC HANGING: Merle Hoffman, manager of an abortion clinic, holds a huge clothes hanger, which she said symbolizes the butchering of women, at a press conference yesterday.

Anger, joy greet abortion ruling

ABORTION Continued from Page 2

that Roe vs. Wade was incorrectly decided and should be reversed," the president added.

Abortion rights advocates were

early as next fall when the justices examine three more abortion cases.

Justice Sandra Day O'Connor, the first woman to ascend to the

Chief Justice William Rehnquist along with Justices Byron White and Anthony Kennedy hinted they were leaning that way.

NOW said it is giving up on the

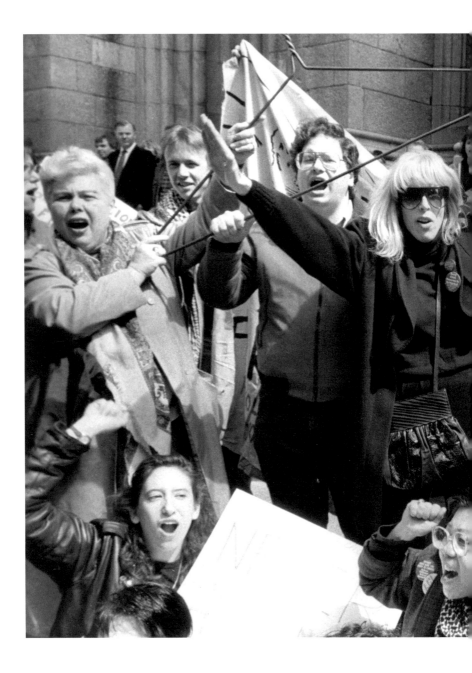

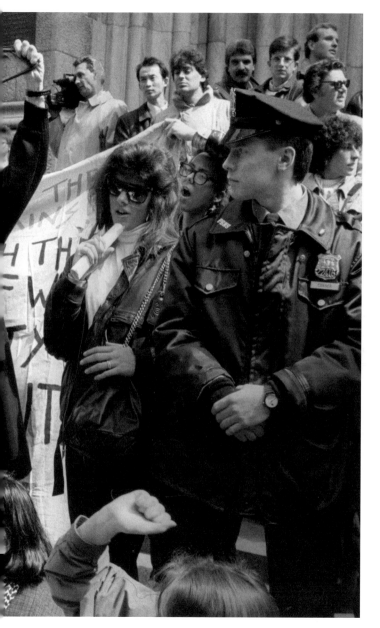

Raising my hanger as a sword at St. Patrick's Cathedral, with members of the New York Pro-Choice Coalition, New York City, 1989.

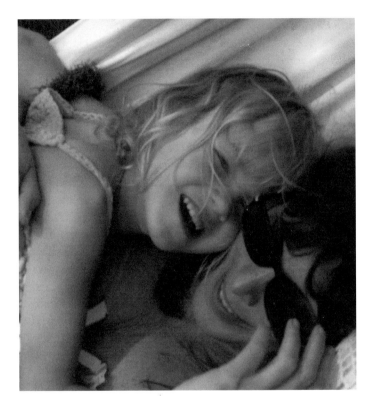

My daughter Sasharina Kate and me at our home in East Hampton,
New York, 2007. PHOTO: KELLY MALLINSON.

What about permanent harm to the mother? In one Washington, DC, case, a pregnant woman dying of cancer was advised by George Washington University Hospital administrators to undergo a cesarean section against her wishes. A local judge ordered the operation to be performed because he felt there was a slight chance of saving the fetus, and the woman was going to die anyway. What would the difference be if she died a few weeks earlier? The cesarean was performed, the woman died, the fetus died, and the operation was listed as a "contributing factor" to her death on her death certificate.

In another well-publicized battle over fetal rights, Nancy Klein, seventeen weeks pregnant, had remained in a coma for two months after a tragic automobile accident. Told by physicians that his wife's life was at risk more and more with each day that the pregnancy developed within her, her husband ordered an abortion. Two right-to-life attorneys, one of whom attempted to become "Baby Klein's" guardian, filed legal brief after legal brief to prevent the life-saving abortion for Nancy. In a radio debate with one of the attorneys, John Broderick, I asked him what he would do if it were his wife's life that hung in the balance. "A baby is a baby is a baby," he said. I have a photo of Bill Baird and me in front of the Suffolk County Court House, the two of us the lone pro-choice demonstrators at the trial.

The rise of fetal rights placed a woman's job, social standing, economic security, and her very life at risk. Right-to-lifers claimed to act in the name of "innocents," for the sake of their human rights, by the order of god. But I viewed fetal rights as a smoke screen, an opaque barrier, an intellectual and imaginative device to control women's lives and reproductive choices. The fetus had become a weapon that could be used against women to reinforce the status quo.

VIOLENCE IS A LANGUAGE, and the antis were becoming more and more articulate. At the encouragement of their leaders the antis began taking their crusade to our clinics, where they could be physically confrontational. Joseph Scheidler of the Pro-Life Action League—the "Green Berets of the Pro-Life Movement"—published a book on how to harass and intimidate abortion providers and clinic patients entitled *Closed: 99 Ways to Stop Abortion*. He quickly became the leader of the activist wing of the anti-abortion movement, bragging that the rate of abortion complications went up when there were demonstrators in front of clinics.

Nineteen eighty-five alone saw approximately 150 attacks against abortion clinics and family planning providers. The newspapers seemed to report a new attack every day. A woman in Brooklyn was violently thrown against the wall of a clinic by an off-duty police officer screaming, "In the name of Jesus, do you know what they are doing inside there?" An eighteen-year-old perpetrator of what were called the "Christmas bombings" against a clinic in Pensacola, Florida, called the blasts a "gift to Jesus on his birthday." In Huntsville, Alabama, a Catholic priest threw red paint into a clinic waiting room and injured two staff members, while "sidewalk counselors" thrust photos of dismembered fetuses in women's faces and screamed that they were "murdering their children." A gunshot shattered the living-room window of Supreme Court Justice Harry Blackmun, the man who wrote the Courts' majority decision legalizing abortion.

Other terrorist-style intimidation methods were even more sinister: a clinic counselor returning home one evening found her cat decapitated. A man drove his war surplus vehicle directly into a clinic, destroying two waiting rooms. Anti-abortionists noted license plate numbers of patients' cars at clinics, used police connections to get their names and phone numbers, and called them in the middle of the night to harass them with a recording of a childish voice crying, "Mommy, mommy, why did you kill me?" This tactic was particularly used against teenagers.

On ABC's *Nightline*, Cal Thomas, spokesperson for the Moral Majority, approved the violence against clinics, which he said would "stir a national debate on abortion." He claimed that the violence was against "bricks and stones"—not people. By denying that the continuous and escalating violence against women's health care centers across the country involved planned and coordinated acts of terrorism, the conservative media, the FBI, and the Reagan Administration callously disregarded women's constitutional rights and fed the fanatical zeal of the terrorists.

God's word was the theory, and bombing clinics and harassing women and doctors was the practice. What we in the pro-choice movement called terrorism, they called battle tactics. Were those who tried to assassinate Hitler and bomb Auschwitz terrorists? Anti-choicers were like today's "freedom fighters" who saw themselves as knights of a higher cause, made even more intense when the cause was a lost one. The womb had become a true battlefield, and we were all soldiers, willing or not.

Each time there was word of another clinic bombing or invasion, each time someone called me Hitler, each day when I walked into Choices past screaming antis and pink plastic fetuses, I travelled further into the trenches. One Monday, a day when many women were there for pre- and post-natal care, Choices received a bomb threat. The male caller allotted us less than fifteen minutes to leave the premises before we'd all be blown up. The call turned out to be a hoax, but that didn't alter the horror we all felt.

I arranged for my staff to work with the Brooklyn Martial Arts Center to learn self-defense. The first thing that was taught was how to scream—an exercise that had to be repeated many times, since women were unused to speaking up and speaking out. My secretary attended a course with the Bureau of Alcohol, Tobacco, and Firearms to learn how to correctly open my mail so that she could avoid damage from a letter bomb. I got used to checking the bottom of my car for bombs and taking different routes to the clinic, looking over my shoulder the whole way.

AMID THE TURMOIL of my days at Choices, my life was changed irrevocably by another kind of opposing force. I received a piece of paper that would hang over the next seven years of my life like the sword of Damocles. It was a subpoena from the Deputy Attorney General for Medicaid Fraud Control announcing that I was being investigated.

HIP's law firm Stroock, Stroock, and Lavan advised me to hire Thomas Puccio, the attorney who defended Claus Von Bulow when he was accused of attempting to murder his wife. This was comparable to using an elephant to swat a fly, and only made the civil servants of the Health Department more incensed.

It took three years before I even learned exactly why they were investigating me, what they considered fraudulent in my practice. Feeling like Joseph K. in Franz Kafka's *The Trial*, I almost went crazy going over and over every act of my professional career at Choices, trying to figure out what exactly could be construed as a felony.

Those years were a special kind of hell. It felt as though I had a terminal disease that would go into remission and rear up again unexpectedly. I never knew when another subpoena would come, when the prosecutors would want another piece of information. At one point there were two grand juries sitting on me and interviewing my employees about the most minute details of my professional life. The boundaries I'd so carefully fostered no longer existed; I was a potential felon, and my employees now held a silent and palpable power over me that I could not even articulate. I had to maintain the image of normalcy—give directives, meet with them, act as if none of it was happening. I could not even allow an unguarded glance to betray me, because if I gave the impression of communicating with them about their testimony, I would be accused of obstructing justice, yet another felony.

Eventually the prosecutor had a meeting with my attorneys and I finally learned the reason for the investigation. Because we were a licensed facility, I saw patients who could not have anesthesia during their procedures because Medicaid didn't cover it. I felt it was unfair that women with private insurance or cash could have greater care and comfort during their procedure than women who were poor, so I decided to offer anesthesia to Medicaid patients for fifty dollars (or whatever they could afford)—much less than it actually cost, but it defrayed the loss a bit. I had patients sign a form outlining the fact that this was not part of their Medicaid coverage and if they chose they could pay what they could afford out of pocket. I finally learned that the Medicaid regulations did not allow providers to charge any out-of-pocket expenses at all to Medicaid recipients; this was considered Medicaid fraud, a felony.

Marty offered to "take the rap" for me, but they wanted me. I told very few people, so he and I were left to ourselves to handle our anxiety. Out of frustration we would attack each other, blame one another for something for which no blame could be placed. We came home from our long days as weary warriors, no energy left over to comfort or actively support each other. Marty began having difficulty concentrating as he grew older. Things started to go badly for him politically within the HIP system. Those in power had to know about the indictment proceedings, because his vulnerability would be theirs. If the wife of the chairman of the Medical Group Council of HIP was indicted for Medicaid fraud, HIP would have to eliminate him; he endangered their own political survival. And of course, Choices would be finished.

IF THERE WAS a possibility of no future, I would throw myself boldly into the present. I embodied Primo Levi's words, "The aims of life are the best defense against death."

I woke at daybreak most mornings to prepare for actions, do radio interviews, or go in to defend my clinic against anti-choice demonstrations. I was becoming increasingly frustrated with what I saw as the passivity of the pro-choice forces. The antis were a passionate, at times dangerous, radical force; the pro-choice movement was reasoned, conscious, political—reserved. That had to change. We'd had some rallies and marches, we'd published articles and made statements, but we were continually on the defensive, and such strategies were usually created pell-mell, quickly, without deep strategic thought or discussion. We were being attacked, and I felt we were just standing there taking it, hoping our problems would right themselves or be reasoned away.

Feminists had to create a collective *J'Accuse*. Any individual woman who stands up against a powerful man must shed her "good girl" mentality to match his aggression. Real resistance, like great social change, doesn't happen just because people get angry. Anger is not enough. We had to say no to the system, no to the historical definitions of "female," and no to the historical oppression of our class. It was time for feminists to match the anger of the antis with our own righteous rage.

In 1985 I volunteered to lead a pro-choice march and rally to commemorate the twelfth anniversary of *Roe*. Members of NARAL and NOW had been talking about marching down Thirty-Fourth Street to the right-to-life headquarters, but no one wanted to lead it. It was dangerous to be so high profile; the rash of threats and bombings had left people afraid to come out.

I was afraid, too, but I knew facing my fear was the only way to practice and display courage.

I dressed carefully the morning of January 22. I knew that the cameras were going to be on me. I wore an Italian trench coat that looked like something out of the late thirties in Berlin. With civil rights attorney William Kunstler standing protectively at my side, I took my place on the platform, raised my bullhorn, and made a great rousing speech to the couple hundred people who had bravely come out for the march.

We rallied and marched with passion that day, but antichoicers had also marched—Nellie Gray led seventy thousand of them in Washington on her annual March for Life. It was obvious that there was a necessity for progressive women and men to work together in coalition. If I could unite the factions of the pro-choice community, emphasize our shared goals and minimize our differences, I could channel our collective energy to pose a formidable challenge to the antis and their political allies. I put out a call for members, sending letters, placing ads, and calling people personally to tell them that it was important that we all meet to strategize and come up with a plan. The enthusiastic response I received led to the founding of the New York Pro-Choice Coalition (PCC), the first umbrella organization of pro-choice individuals, politicians, nonprofits, activists, providers, and organizations committed to ensuring legal, safe abortion in New York.[16] Our mission statement held that we would fully utilize the talents and input of organizations and individuals to ensure the continued existence of reproductive freedom for all women.

This was, of course, easier said than done. I found myself once again the leader of a group of people with very different ideas about how things should be run and how our goals should be accomplished. We agreed that it was necessary to come up with a new strategy to combat the language, symbols, and actions of the antis. The question was, could we agree on the tactics?

One of our first internal debates revolved around how to publicly counter the imagery used by the pro-lifers. We had to find a psychological match for those shameless bloody fetuses, contrasted with the "cute" pairs of fetal feet. The possibility of using the iconic image of Gerri Santoro—she bled to death as a result of a botched self-abortion in 1964—lying dead in a pool of blood was brought up, but quickly put aside for fear it would be seen as just another exploitative media image. The use of multiethnic and multigenerational women's faces was also discussed as a variation of NARAL's theme, "We are your mothers, your sisters, your daughters, your friends," but it was felt that this was too timid a response.

Finally, I suggested we use the simple image of the wire coat hanger, which represented all of the awful homegrown abortion remedies: poison, lye, throwing oneself down the stairs, putting a knife in one's stomach. It addressed the severity of the issue without stooping to graphic shock tactics. Many thought it was too negative, and some representatives of Planned Parenthood worried that it might turn off funders. Others thought that young people would not know what it meant. Since we were unable to reach a consensus, I went ahead and used the hanger as a symbol myself. It went on to become a ubiquitous symbol of reproductive rights and a powerful visual cue that reached younger women.

The lack of minority representation within the PCC was another subject of many heated discussions. We broadly publicized our meetings and were totally open to new membership, but few women of color joined us. This meant that when women of color did attend, they were often put in the uncomfortable position of speaking for their entire racial group.

Another source of tension within the PCC was more personally directed at me. I'd founded the coalition on the strength of my will and ideas, and I was the natural leader for practical reasons as well: thanks to Choices, I was able to spend a great deal of money supporting the coalition's political actions—and many of the activists on an individual basis, too. Some saw this as contradictory; I was radical on the streets, but I had the financial resources to assist in the necessary day-to-day needs of street politics: having expensive props made, paying for printing costs, phone bills, transportation, and publicity. People were grateful for my generosity, but there was always some degree of resentment. Rhonda Copelon, a fellow activist who would become a lifelong friend and supporter, once called me a mixed bag.

Others—socialists, in particular—were sensitive to the notion of me or anyone being the acknowledged leader of the coalition. I recall one telling occurrence that took place during an action in front of the New York City Planned Parenthood: when the police asked, "Who is the leader here?" I had to carefully reply, "I can speak for the group." I was able to understand everyone's need for recognition and participation.

These tensions were the predictable result of forming a coalition, but they never came close to overpowering the success of PCC as an organization. Working together, certain of our common goal, the coalition proved itself to be one of the most formidable opponents of the anti-choice movement. Over the next few years feminists across the country were beginning to recognize that all kinds of silences had to be broken. Wide media coverage of rallies, marches, and awareness weeks—on both sides of the war—placed the abortion debate more prominently in the public spotlight than ever.

Every January tens of thousands of antis marched on Washington, vowing to overturn *Roe v. Wade*. Reagan offered his support with statements like "Together we will insure that the resources of government are not used to promote or perform abortions."[17] The PCC and other pro-choice organizations answered them with meticulously organized rallies of our own that meshed performance, battle, and theater. In one of our first actions, the PCC participated in the nationwide commemoration of the anniversary of *Roe v. Wade* with local demonstrations in ninety-seven cities. Women lobbied to defend and broaden the right to choose abortion and birth control; some delivered coat hangers to right-wing legislators.[18]

Our New York contingent was five hundred strong, and together we chanted:

> Not the Church,
> Not the State,
> Women must decide our fate.
>
> Not only a mother,
> Not only a wife
> A woman's life is a human life.
>
> Gay, straight, black, white
> Abortion is a woman's right!

"Women should be able to have abortions without the threat of dying by bombing or terrorist attack," I told *Newsday* that afternoon.

Each action required dozens of meetings and hours of planning. There were dates, venues, and speakers to work out, each element carefully orchestrated to make the maximum impact. I often took on the role of emcee and gave the opening speech.

I began our 1986 rally in Bryant Park by asking for a moment of silence for all the women who had laid down their lives for the right to choose. I asked those who had had an abortion or knew someone who had to raise their hands, and as each hand raised it was as if we were being validated again and again. Some shot up boldly, others came up more slowly—but each one was a triumph of will.

Time for me was measured by planning, actions, and political events. There were no babies' birthdays to celebrate; my husband's birthdays were more of a reminder of his mortality and my potential loss than anything else; and I was so totally immersed in the work that January 22, the anniversary of *Roe v. Wade*, began to take on as much, and sometimes more, significance as March 6, my own birthday. I felt as if I had been born for this moment in history, that the dreams of my girlhood had finally come to life, and my work was a continual affirmation of that.

MY WORK WITH the PCC led to some of my deepest friendships. I met Phyllis Chesler at a demonstration for Mary Beth Whitehead in Hackensack, New Jersey, in 1987. Whitehead was fighting to gain custody over a baby she'd contractually arranged to carry to term for a wealthy woman, making her the baby's surrogate mother. The court conducted a "best interest of the child" analysis to determine which woman had the right to raise the child, putting definitions of motherhood in the spotlight. When I learned that Whitehead had been declared an "unfit mother" for giving her daughter pots and pans to play with instead of stuffed animals, I decided to go down to the courthouse for her trial.

Phyllis had convened a group of women to rally for Whitehead's right to keep her daughter. Watching her give a passionate speech in front of an empty crib, I was immediately drawn to her fierce support of Whitehead. I introduced myself to her after the speech and told her I wanted to cover her cause for my magazine.

She thanked me and asked me to get her a cold drink from inside.

The next day I shocked her by sending her a thousand-dollar check to support her work. I knew that she was considered brilliant and controversial—she had written the feminist classic *Women and Madness*—and I also knew that she saw herself as a prophet and a revolutionary, and was comfortable working alone. We had much in common.

We slowly became friends. We both wanted and craved action, and being romantics with vivid imaginations, we began to make plans for creating a feminist world. Once we placed an ad in the *Village Voice* recruiting feminist warriors: THE FEMINIST GOVERNMENT NEEDS YOU! We envisioned a kind of feminist guardian angel brigade that would patrol the streets of New York City insuring the safety of women, stopping domestic violence and sexual harassment, and defending patients at abortion clinics. We received only two responses, so that dream had to be put on hold.

Phyllis was also unusual in the world of the radical feminist leadership in that she was a single mother choosing to bring her son Ariel up to be an active part of her political life. I remember her defining rape for him at my kitchen table when he was just nine years old. She took him with us to some pro-choice rallies, and he later worked at Choices for a couple of summers. We all occasionally spent time at Kate Millett's farm during her famous celebrations of the Japanese festival Obon, sharing her wonderful feminist arcadia.

Andrea Dworkin was another dedicated feminist with whom I became friends through my work as a pro-choice leader and publisher of the magazine. She, too, cast a very large shadow. Andrea was always soft-spoken, smiling through her small talk until she came to her reality—then she became a fiery herald of truth.

I was always impressed by her work against rape and pornography, especially her ability to put theory into practice, as in 1983 when she and Catharine MacKinnon were hired by the Minneapolis city government to draft an antipornography civil rights ordinance (which would define pornography as a civil rights violation and allow those harmed by the industry to sue for damages) as an amendment to the City of Minneapolis civil rights ordinance.

In a sense she was the Robespierre of the movement. This analogy came to life when Andrea reacted to *A Book of Women's Choices: Abortion, Menstrual Extraction, RU-486*, which Carol Downer had written with Rebecca Chalker detailing ways that women could sabotage potential anti-abortion laws, one of which was to claim that they had been raped. Andrea felt very strongly that if women were to fake rapes as a tactic in the struggle to access legal abortion, it would denude and diminish her work fighting rape and violence against women. She called Downer a traitor to the movement and told me over the phone that if she had the power, she would have her executed. I asked whether she would like a guillotine to be put up in the town square for this purpose and she found the idea quite pleasing.

AS MY CIRCLE OF FRIENDS broadened and my professional reputation grew, I had the opportunity to exchange ideas with some of the most brilliant and unique political and literary women of the time: Petra Kelly, Florynce Kennedy, Kate Millett, Erica Jong, and so many others. I wanted our life-altering conversations and ideas to reach past our meetings, our speeches, and even our publications. *On the Issues* was a success as far as radical non-mainstream feminist publications can be called successful—at its height we had twenty thousand subscribers nationally and internationally—but I wanted to reach more people, to be on the cutting edge. With the right medium we could spark public dialogue on subjects that were too often passed over in the mainstream media. And the way to reach mass audiences was not through print magazines; it was on television.

In 1986, I decided to create, coproduce, and host a feminist talk show I called *MH: On the Issues*. It was a series of ten thirty-minute cable shows syndicated to eleven million homes: the first feminist show on television.

I interviewed Bella Abzug, Bill Baird, Carol Bellamy, Susie Orbach, Elizabeth Holtzman, and NOW NY chapter president Jennifer Brown. I celebrated my fortieth birthday on the air with Deborah Perry—a self-described feminist witch—who blew bubbles for me and gave me two presents: a small candle from Gloria Steinem's fiftieth birthday cake, and a large multicolored candle in the shape of a vagina.

Betty Friedan, on the other hand, was known as a kind of sacred monster—some called her the "mother of the women's movement"—and she had a reputation for being difficult at best. On the date of her guest appearance the cab that we sent for her was late, prompting her to call from her apartment screaming that we were all a bunch of idiots and she had no time for this. She finally capitulated and we all waited with baited breath for her to arrive at the studio. One young assistant, so very excited to meet her, held a dog-eared copy of *The Feminine Mystique* on her lap ready to be autographed.

In walked Betty muttering and bellowing, "Let's get this fucking thing started—I can only stay for twenty minutes." She rushed past that young girl without even noticing her.

Throughout the interview Betty was in a state of high anxiety, glancing at her watch and fidgeting, until finally she interrupted a question I was posing to say, "I'm very sorry, but I must leave now." She got up from her chair, dragging her microphone behind her, and stormed out of the studio while the cameras kept rolling. I continued with the show, having another ten minutes to fill.

FOR SOME WOMEN feminism is a way of seeing the world more clearly, of taking off the glasses that society, culture, and geography have placed upon you. The best of them had an "aristocracy of the soul" because of their work and their vision for women's freedom, and even though this did not always translate into altered behavior, I made allowances for them most of the time, as I am sure they felt they made allowances for me. I was attracted to thinkers who were able to bridge the gap between theory and practice, to leap the distance from radical writings to the soapbox to the streets. We were feminists engaged in a just war sharing the privilege of a critical consciousness, and we knew we had to support each other's missions and lend one another our strengths.

This truth bolstered my political and professional life, but the knowledge that I could lose my business for Medicaid fraud, which I hid from almost all of my friends, never ceased to haunt me during those years. My possible indictment still felt like an impending death sentence, a terrible secret I had to keep. I remember sitting in my office and looking at my political posters, saying a kind of private goodbye.

Unlike Marty, who could find release and forgetting in sleep, I was tortured with anxiety at night. I realized that just as he had his defense mechanisms, I would have to develop mine.

In the midst of my crisis I was fortunate to meet Mahin Hassibi, a well-known child psychiatrist. I was immediately attracted to this small black-haired Iranian woman. I soon found she was the most well read of any person I had ever known and the only one who had ever completed Kant's *Critique of Pure Reason*, Gibbon's *History of the Decline and Fall of the Roman Empire*, and all of Proust, both in French and English.

Hers was a political experience of a very different kind: she had participated in the Iranian Revolution, as an activist in the streets and as a doctor treating other activists who had their heads broken open by the Shah's goons. A close friend of hers had set herself on fire in Tehran to protest women's status in that country.[19] The power struggle between the Americans and the Iranians over the years meant that she, too, was a pariah of sorts in American society. She was harassed in Metropolitan Hospital, where she was the assistant director of child psychiatry, by being called "Khomeini's daughter." Over time she became a true soul mate, a woman who was always there to talk and help center me. We would have hours of philosophical conversations that gave me a kind of pleasure that nothing else could and distracted me from my troubles at the clinic.

After seven years, many thousands of dollars, and much psychological trauma, a legal way out was found to finally satisfy the prosecutors without having Choices ruined or myself indicted. Because the infraction had happened while Choices was still operating as Flushing Women's Medical Center, Dr.

Leo Orris (who had been part owner then) agreed to help us plead guilty in this case under our old name. And since Flushing Women's Medical Center no longer technically existed as such, Choices as it now existed was saved from destruction.

The end of my nightmare was reported in an article published on the front page of the *New York Law Journal* on December 28, 1988: "A Queens abortion clinic pleaded guilty yesterday in state court to illegally overcharging 400 Medicaid patients and paid $50,000 in restitution." A relatively small price to pay in the end; the hardest part was to accept this verdict as the last word. Clearly, it wasn't.

I was sued again soon afterward by a pro-life doctor, Cordelia Beverly, in what turned out to be a major commercial free speech case. Choices had been publishing and freely distributing calendars celebrating reproductive rights since 1980. In 1988 we illustrated the month of June with a picture taken at the Third Regional Conference of Women in Medicine that depicted Dr. Cordelia Beverly posing with Dr. Lena Edwards, an award-winning physician, both in attendance there. The inclusion of Dr. Beverly's picture was meant to be an honor, but she felt we had put her life at risk by publicly associating her with an abortion clinic. She held that Choices had illegally used her image as an advertisement.

By vote of 3–1 the court affirmed partial summary judgment on Dr. Beverly's claim under Civil Rights Law 51. The case, which centered on whether my giving out free calendars nationally was advertising or education, made the front page of the *Law Journal*. After that I was very careful to get appropriate consent before I printed anyone's photos, especially if it pertained to Choices.

DEALING WITH THESE ANXIETIES and obstacles made me more sensitive than ever to the discrimination and pain that marked so many of my patient's lives. The little girls and adolescents with wide eyes expressing what could not be spoken still got to me the most. I wanted to protect them, to give them their own defense mechanisms that would enable them to move through these difficult years without becoming casualties of the sexual culture. Parental consent was a hot topic at the time, thanks to Reagan's attempt to pass a law that would require federally funded programs to notify parents when their children requested services. When I first opened my clinic I supported parental consent, thinking it best to have the support of a committed adult when making such a hard decision. But the 1988 case of Becky Bell, an Indiana teenager who died as a result of an illegal abortion she had sought rather than tell her parents she was pregnant, showed what could go wrong if minors were prohibited from making their own choices.

When I was asked to give the first family planning and birth control talk (called "What Will Mama Say?") to the Girl Scouts of the USA chapter in New York City, I was excited to have the opportunity to reach girls before they were faced with such a life-altering choice. I was amazed at how ignorant the girls were about their bodies and sex. They were so open and trusting, sharing with us their questions and fears. One girl revealed that she'd been sexually abused by a relative. Another asked the question, "Can you get pregnant from kissing?" Later the PCC sponsored a well-advertised Teen Speakout on Choice, at which I hosted a panel of experts who could answer the teenagers' questions about their reproductive rights: whether they wanted to have an abortion, keep the baby, or give it up for adoption.

The Creedmoor Mental Health Players, a group of talented staff from Creedmoor State Hospital, heard about my program with the Girl Scouts and asked if I'd be interested in collaborating with them to hold a workshop series at Rikers Island Prison. As we talked with the male and female inmates on subjects like battered women, rape, alcoholism, depression, and sexual issues, I found that I had a connection to the prisoners. I was interested in women who were in prison for crossing boundaries, women who killed their abusers, or women behind bars for political reasons.

Meanwhile I noticed another underserved, shamed group that was being overlooked and discriminated against when it came to health care. Lesbians tended to visit their gynecologists much less frequently then heterosexual women, unwilling because of the medical assumption of heterosexuality. They were given medical forms questioning their use of birth control, their "marital status," and so on; there was absolutely no conception of the need for sex education and health care directed toward women without men.

I made sure that my staff knew how to be sensitive to the needs of lesbians so that Choices would be a safe space for them to seek care. But the obstacles homosexuals faced extended far beyond the boundaries of the clinic, so when I heard about the story of Karen Thompson, a lesbian whose lover, Sharon Kowalski, was in a car accident that left her a quadriplegic and unable to speak, I knew I had to help publicize it. Because Sharon's parents refused to recognize the fact that their daughter was a lesbian, they barred Karen from visiting Sharon's treatment facility. Karen was traveling the country, trying to set up interviews and give speeches to enlist support for what had become her crusade. She was fighting for the rights of all LGBT individuals. When I broke her story in *On the Issues* in 1987, Karen hadn't seen her partner in two years.

Gay men were dealing with a new health crisis around this time. I had covered AIDS in the first issue of my magazine in

1982 when it was an inchoate threat; by 1986, it was exploding like the abortion issue had ten years before. And like abortion, it was controversial, dangerous, and profound. AIDS had become the gay man's unwanted pregnancy. For the first time since penicillin eliminated the fear of venereal disease, men were facing potentially life-threatening results from sex, an issue with which women had always had to grapple.

When I visited the AIDS ward at San Francisco General, I saw that the disease had galvanized the gay community and changed the conventional avenues of medical treatment. I thought of my beginnings at Choices in the early seventies, before abortion had been legalized nationally, when we still dealt with all the shame, guilt, fear, and stigma. I remembered how the community of women had reached out—how they referred, educated, counseled, and supported women seeking abortions. In the case of AIDS, where medical technology had not been able to develop a definitive test to diagnose, let alone treat the disease, physicians so used to playing god had to face the reality of limited answers. Now, as then, the medical community had out of necessity stepped aside for love, for another definition of healing. This was Patient Power.

Pregnant teens, women in prison, lesbians, gays—they were all pariahs, and they were all suffering, even dying, from the resulting guilt and shame that status produced. Shame was used as a defense by some to not seek services, and by others to block out possible help from the outside. And as with abortion, situations branded as transgressive or even illegal prevented many people from forming connections and political coalitions to address their rights. Many cast-outs experienced a kind of existential disgust that caused them to deny or ignore their reality. But the battle cry of the AIDS movement—that Silence=Death—said it all.

IN THE LATE 1980S, another front opened in the war against women. In 1986 Randall Terry had founded Operation Rescue, an organization whose initial tactics involved peaceful sit-in demonstrations at abortion clinics inspired by the civil rights demonstrations led by Dr. King in the 1960s. But soon Terry and his protesters progressed to more violent tactics, shutting down a clinic in Cherry Hill, New Jersey. Operation Rescue sprang to prominence as a national organization during the 1988 Democratic National Convention in Atlanta, Georgia, where hundreds of demonstrators were arrested, capturing national attention. By then they had adopted a slogan to fit the times: "If you believe abortion is murder, act like it's murder." That year, Reagan gave a speech to more than fifty thousand pro-life supporters gathered in Washington to mourn fifteen years of *Roe v. Wade*. "We're told about a woman's right to control her own body, but doesn't an unborn child have a higher right, and that is to life, liberty, and the pursuit of happiness?" he asked.

In April of 1988, Operation Rescue summoned its ranks to New York City to begin what they called "a righteous, peaceful uprising of god-fearing people across the country that will 'inspire' politicians to correct man's law, and make child-killing illegal again. . . . If we don't end this holocaust very soon, the judgment of god is going to fall on this nation." Hundreds came to New York with the intention of gathering in large numbers to blockade abortion clinics across New York City over the course of several days. Their goal was to get favorable media coverage and project the image of a groundswell of pious people against abortion while preventing women from exercising their reproductive rights.

I led the PCC on the offensive. We declared a Reproductive Freedom Week that would kick off with a march and rally on Friday, April 29, the day before Operation Rescue arrived in New York City. Approximately fifteen hundred people participated in our march, the largest pro-choice event in New York in ten years. Leading the way, I walked up to the right-to-life office clutching a "Support Operation Rescue" placard in my hands. I held it up to the crowd and tore it to pieces, declaring my action a symbol of how women were going fight back against the terrorists in Operation Rescue.

Marches were always an important public statement of support. They gave people who otherwise would not get involved an opportunity to get into the streets and show their support for choice. Women could bring their mothers, daughters, and friends to bond over the issues in the exhilarating, almost celebratory atmosphere created by thousands of people coming together for a common cause. But it was the persistent, grueling, day-to-day activism that was necessary to resist the conservative and oppressive forces of the Right. We had to make sure a band of soldiers was present at every clinic, every day, to physically ensure that women's rights weren't blocked by the antis.

The PCC meeting space turned into a war room. We began by writing and distributing a pamphlet called "The Battle to Defend Abortion Clinics," the only strategic military pamphlet of the pro-choice movement. It detailed the politics of the battle and included concrete tactical suggestions for organizing against planned and unplanned pro-life demonstrations and actions. The week before Operation Rescue's demonstration we held a training session on how to protect and defend the clinics. People living near the hotels where Operation Rescue activists planned to stay were leafleted and encouraged to give Operation Rescue a "fitting welcome."

For the next week we organized clinic watches and phone trees, dispatching people to the sights Operation Rescue was targeting. We secretly followed Operation Rescue members to find out which clinic they would target next, communicating the information to each other using walkie-talkies. Emergency announcements were made on a radio station (WBAI), giving the location of the facility being attacked and calling on people to come and defend it. Despite our efforts, Operation Rescue succeeded in closing facilities three out of the four days it staged blockades.

So began a long year of defending abortion rights against Operation Rescue.

Many of my mornings in 1988 began at dawn, when the lights of the city mingled with the sunrise. On one such morning I waited with other pro-choice warriors in front of the Carter Hotel, where the troops of Operation Rescue were gathering to begin their terror tactics against a local abortion clinic. Someone handed me a token for the subway, and before I knew it I was swept underground. Then we were running down Twenty-Third Street next to Randall Terry and his cohorts, determined to beat them to the clinic so we could keep those doors open. Terry and I locked eyes and gave each other a nonverbal acknowledgement of our competition as we raced each other down the street.

We did manage to get to those doors, but Terry controlled all the outside traffic. No one could enter or leave, and seeing patients that day was impossible. But by 11 a.m. we were still there, refusing to surrender the clinic to Operation Rescue. Surrounded by their voices singing "Amazing Grace," we chanted, "Not the Church, not the State, women must decide their fate," and "Operation Rescue your name's a lie, you don't care if women die!" I can say them in my sleep even now.

Another day, I was called to assist Eastern Women's Center in the middle of an attack by Operation Rescue. The antis were lying on the floor forming a "Kryptonite Block," a madly creative device that allowed a group of protesters to attach themselves to specially designed bicycle locks that defied police attempts to free them. By the time I arrived at the clinic, five Operation Rescue participants had been in the same positions, leg to neck to ankle to thigh, for approximately three hours; it would be at least another two before the police could dismantle them. One Catholic priest, attached to five women, was sitting with his neck chained like a dog, screaming to the women in the waiting room, "Go home, go home. There'll be no baby killing here today. You will not be killing your babies this Saturday."

They held their biggest action yet on our turf on January 15, 1989. Defying a federal judge's orders to stop blocking clinic entrances, eight hundred Operation Rescue members were arrested during protests at abortion clinics in New York, New Orleans, and Cincinnati. Demonstrators chained themselves together and to fences in front of the clinics, halted elevators, triggered fire alarms, and lay in front of police buses attempting to carry them away. They began their demonstration just as the US Supreme Court agreed to hear an appeal that would have made the fetus a constitutional person with rights and privileges. New York City, the abortion capital of the United States, was to be the place where their national revolution would begin.

In reaction, I arranged for the PCC to hold a "back alley" press conference in an alley between Broadway and Lafayette Streets in Manhattan to emphasize what women would face if the antis were successful in making abortions illegal. I held up my hanger and declared, "As I stand here in this alley among this garbage, this graffiti, this filth and debris, I know that I am possibly standing in and looking at my future—the future of millions of American women. . . . Making abortion illegal will not stop abortion. What it will do is send women by the hundreds of thousands into alleys just like this one.

When that time comes there will be not enough alleys, not enough hospital emergency rooms, and not enough coffins to hold them."

WE FEMINISTS were encouraging the formation of new coalitions and inspiring others to act, or at least think about action. We never let an attack go unanswered, a clinic undefended. But what I wanted was for the entire pro-choice silent majority of the country to stand up and say, women's rights are human rights! We will not allow any of these terrorists to stop our mothers, daughters, sisters, and friends from being able to exercise their moral and constitutional rights. I wanted mass mobilization. A girl can dream, can't she?

This frustration was occupying my mind when an Operation Rescue activist asked, "Where are your troops, Hoffman?" on yet another rainy, cold morning of protesting.

I turned to face my questioner. Middle-aged, white, male, polyester suit, fetal feet button—in all, a good soldier of the Lord.

"Where are your troops?"

I looked past him to our small band of about fifty feminist activists, chanting and intense; beyond the five hundred or so kneeling, praying "rescuers"; past the police, the press, the passersby, and thought about his question. Where were my troops? We appeared sadly outnumbered. Compared to the antis, we always were.

The small, two-story abortion clinic under attack was situated between Third and Lexington Avenues. As the drama unfolded, business went on as usual. Dogs got walked, some people shopped, some stopped to chat, others rushed on to work, all going about their daily routines as if a war were not happening in front of them. My questioner had verbalized one of my private intellectual dialogues. But it was really not so private after all. The question of just where the feminist movement was now, where the feminist movement was going, whether the feminist movement was alive or dead, had become a popular issue around which media, politicians, and anyone who felt like it could instantly pontificate.

Of course the "rescuer" had a far more literal interpretation of this question in mind. He was merely counting heads.

Operation Rescue was bent on trying to publicly project the image of a groundswell of pious people against abortion through the media, and at this it was somewhat effective. It chose as its battlefront small, unprotected doctors' offices rather than large well-known (and well-prepared) facilities. Considering that every day in New York City alone there were hundreds of women who terminated their pregnancies at any one of at least one hundred providers, Operation Rescue's claim that they were on the way to eliminating abortion was more than slightly exaggerated.

It reminded me of their other exaggerations and falsehoods: their shameless self-comparisons to the likes of Martin Luther King, Jr., or their obscene claim that their movement was akin to the great civil rights struggle of the sixties.

Many people bought their lies. During the reign of Reagan, "double-think" had become the accepted form of social and political reality. Nuclear missiles were "peacekeepers," ketchup was a "vegetable," and all Americans were "better off now" than they had been some time in the past. This sinister tactic of obscuring truth with wishful thinking was actively appropriated by much of the local and national press, which helped Operation Rescue and its participants by affording them a great deal of coverage and sometimes even positive reviews. Reagan himself met personally with Joseph Scheidler and publicly praised him, officially giving these terrorists the highest institutional backing.

The New York City police, many of whom seemed to be politically inclined to Operation Rescue's philosophy, were also caught up in the fantasy. Pursuing a policy of "selective enforcement," police treated the anti-choice blockaders with kid gloves, using stretchers to take protesters away gently, issuing desk tickets, and releasing Operation Rescue "prisoners of war" soon afterward, allowing them to return to the blockade site once again.

This treatment was in marked contrast to that given pro-choice activists, who were pushed, pummeled, and herded into small areas behind barricades. It took intense and pressured meetings with Police Commissioner Benjamin Ward to publicly shame the police into upholding the law and ensuring women's access to constitutionally protected medical treatment. Going up against Operation Rescue, we faced the daily possibility of being physically hurt or killed. I almost got clubbed by police in one of the early actions outside of a doctor's office in Queens.

Operation Rescue had succeeded in casting pro-choice forces as the generic "female": dangerous, assertive, selfish, shrill feminists who had to be controlled and diminished if only, at this point, by paper tigers in the press declaring feminism dead and obscuring the progress we made with each march, the successes we had each time we kept a clinic open.

That anti-choice man's question—where are your troops? —helped clarify what I already knew that day. Looking through his eyes, people might have agreed that the right wing was winning. It was an illusion. Yes, we were outnumbered on the streets, and that could be frustrating. But a mass mobilization of sorts *was* occurring. The historic bifurcation between abortion providers and political activists had finally begun to dissolve, and a powerful new alliance was beginning to form. Participation in direct action against Operation

Rescue at clinic sites put ideological feminists face to face with the reality of abortion. Over one million women each year were having legal abortions at clinics across the country, and they each risked harassment, violence, and restrictive, even dangerous, regulations in upcoming Supreme Court cases. Providers were now at the forefront of the abortion rights struggle, and patients themselves, in the midst of the most personal and intimate of decisions and life events, were thrust into a vortex of politics and passion.

Some were reluctant warriors, engaging with the struggle but still unable to own their choice. Others were able to draw strength and courage from the news of pro-choice rallies and actions. Still others marched in the streets, lay down in acts of civil disobedience, wrote checks to pro-choice organizations, or activated students on campuses. Millions more voted only for candidates who expressed the pro-choice position.

We had always had plenty of troops in this battle. They were everywhere, and they were far from outnumbered. They just had to be activated.

I DECIDED IT WAS TIME to make a statement that could not be ignored or manipulated by the media, Reagan, or Operation Rescue. We would deliver a message to the cardinal of New York, John J. O'Connor—a proclamation, a Bill of Rights on abortion. Invoking Luther's *95 Theses* at Wittenberg, we would hold our demands for women's moral, legal, and civil rights to reproductive freedom up on the walls of St. Patrick's Cathedral.

The PCC quietly spread the word to gather across the street from the cathedral on the morning of Sunday, April 2. We gave no further instructions for fear that Operation Rescue would get wind of the plan and stage an opposing action.

I was very careful not to organize the protest at the time of Mass; we would begin just as the service ended.

When the day arrived, everything was in place. As people began pouring forth from the cathedral, pro-choice activists marched across the street to the concrete steps. Mary Lou Greenberg and Maria Lyons stood in front of the massive bronze doors and unfurled a proclamation:

On behalf of the women of New York City and their sisters throughout this country and out of love for the truth and the desire to bring it to light.

We stand here today to affirm the following to Cardinal John J. O'Connor who has blessed, praised, and hosted the anti-abortion fanatics of "Operation Rescue":

That you have consistently turned a deaf ear and a cold heart to women by repeatedly ignoring urgent requests to meet with us about the terrorism and violence towards women that "Operation Rescue" represents.

That you have added to the atmosphere of fear, terror, and anxiety that women must face when attempting to exercise their constitutional right to an abortion.

That you have encouraged the fanaticism and women hating that feeds the politics of "Operation Rescue."

Now, therefore, we stand here not as beggars at your gate but as people of conscience to affirm that:

1. Women are full moral agents with the right and ability to choose when and whether or not they will be mothers.
2. Abortion is a choice made by each individual for profound personal reasons that no man nor state should judge.
3. The right to make reproductive choices is women's legacy throughout history and belongs to every woman regardless of age, class, race, religion, or sexual preference.

4. Abortion is a life-affirming act chosen within the context of women's realities, women's lives, and women's sexuality.

5. Abortion is often the most moral choice in a world that frequently denies health care, housing, education, and economic survival.

Cheering exuberantly and waving coat hangers, hundreds of pro-choice supporters who had been waiting across the street surged to the steps of the cathedral. They began chanting slogans in support of our proclamation. William Kunstler, Charlotte Bunch, Phyllis Chesler (and her son Ariel), Sue Davis, Lawrence Lader, Joan Gibbs, Rhonda Copelon, and Esperanza Martell were among the crowd.

I made my way up the church steps with the six-foot hanger I had commissioned for the occasion. It was a symbol of potential terror and aggression against all women, but it was also the symbol of our future. And taking my place in front of the doors to the cathedral, I knew that it was also the ultimate symbol of both defiance and gentle desecration.

As I lifted the hanger above my head, the crowed throbbed and screamed with new energy. Police officers showed up on the scene, pushed our people back across the street, and arrested nine activists for trespassing on church property, resisting arrest, and disorderly conduct. We marched after them with Norman Siegel of the New York Civil Liberties Union to the precinct to rescue our activists.

The media could not ignore this one. It was our most successful, best publicized action yet, covered in every major newspaper across the United States. The *New York Times* quoted me on the cover of the Metro Section, saying, "Women's rights are in a state of emergency," and the *Philadelphia*

Enquirer marked the occasion as "an important strategic change in the movement." It was the first time pro-choice supporters had been arrested. Some of them had planned to be. Others had been caught up in the intense spirit of the moment, ready for a higher level of sacrifice. We had placed our thesis on the great doors of the cathedral, where statues of the saints looked coldly at the passing activity below them. It was a time of radicalism, a moment when the light pointed to the root cause and we addressed it.

The Russian Front

"As a woman I have no country. . . .
As a woman my country is the whole world."
—VIRGINIA WOOLF

By the late 1980s I'd had my hand in almost every the-ater of the war for reproductive rights, including legal, political, medical, academic, media, activist, and personal spheres. As Reagan's conservative reign came to an end, I felt the need to get involved in yet another: electoral politics, one of the most important battlegrounds in our struggle. This arena was all about compromise and strategy; it was time for me to get pragmatic.

As a leader of the pro-choice movement I'd had the chance to see the political scene firsthand. Many politicians who had started their careers as allies with high personal standards were forced to make compromises to stay in the game. Marty would politick at dinners and meetings, and back at home he'd tell me what he really thought of those bastards, warn-ing me to "trust no one," a lesson I was learning quite well on my own. Though I'd decided not to go into politics myself, I understood the importance of working with politicians. I was constantly attending fundraisers and meeting with pro-choice supporters, pushing my agenda with my hand always ready to sign a check. Often the best I could do was whatever it took to get the least bad candidate elected and the needed bills vetoed or passed.

At one elegant Upper East Side fundraiser I met Oregon senator Bob Packwood, an early and ardent player in the abortion rights struggle, a staunch and able ally of the pro-choice forces on the Republican side of the Senate. Our connection was so immediate that I solicited and received a piece from him for *On the Issues*, after which he called me to request a meeting at a New York City hotel.

We discussed the existential nature of power, the causes for which we'd be willing to die, those for which we would be willing to send others to die. He seemed to be genuinely moved by the responsibilities of his office and the loneliness of power. Even with the intensity of our conversation and the compliments he interspersed throughout our time together, I did not expect his embrace and attempted French kiss in the middle of Park Avenue as I hailed a cab.

Of course I did not believe that men who did good deeds in the public arena were necessarily good boys in private. Packwood's sexual come-on was just that; the fact that it was more an adolescent groping than a sophisticated seduction was, to me, more of an annoyance than a threat. But as the world later found out, Packwood had been sexually harassing women on his staff since at least 1975. He was eventually forced to resign from office under threat of expulsion. A piece in the *New York Times* described the fire against him by women's groups as being fueled by a sense of betrayal. Was Packwood's early support of abortion rights, it asks, a true expression of avant-garde Republican liberalism, or a form of political opportunism?

Without Packwood's influence the pro-choice position

would have had less representation in the Senate, and I was willing to overlook his indiscretion with me for the sake of my greater cause. Working in the sphere of politics meant interacting with very strange bedfellows; however, I wasn't sorry when he was caught.

As the leader of the PCC, I had political agency, too. Abortion was especially hot the year of the 1989 New York City mayoral race due to the passage of *Webster v. Reproductive Health Services*, a Supreme Court ruling allowing states the right to limit access to abortions. New York was still the "abortion capital of the nation," and the issue was being watched carefully for its impact on this election.

The PCC used our high profile to make abortion one of the defining issues of the race. Before the primaries we sent out a questionnaire to the candidates, both Republicans and Democrats, detailing the nuances of a truly pro-choice position and asking them where they fell on the spectrum. We used their answers to rate them on a scale of one to ten.

The race was a heated one, with Edward Koch defending his seat in the primaries against Manhattan Borough President David Dinkins as well as two other candidates. The winner would run against Rudolph Giuliani. Our ratings of the candidates—seven in all—had the potential to play a big role in the outcome of the election. We planned to hold a press conference a few weeks before the primaries to broadcast our results.

When we analyzed and rated the questionnaires, Dinkins scored slightly higher than Koch, who had made deals with the archdiocese that we felt betrayed the movement. Dinkins was the favorite among the progressives and a majority of the PCC, so publicizing him as our top pick was seen as a given.

On the sweltering summer night before the press conference I received an urgent call from Howard Rubenstein's office. Someone had gotten wind that the pro-choice coalition would be exhibiting Koch's large photo underneath Dinkins's on the eight-by-twelve-foot "choice chart" we had created for the press. Rubenstein summoned me to his office to let me know in no uncertain terms that if Dinkins were rated higher then Koch (whom Rubenstein was representing) it might cost him the race.

Howard was someone with whom I had worked for many years. I'd strategized the Patient Power campaign with him, and his son had worked with me on all of my political actions. Now here he was, sitting in his glass tower office with a couple of Koch's aides and laying the responsibility of the outcome of the mayoral race on me!

I was receiving my honorary doctorate in compromise. After a practically sleepless night during which I conferred with the PCC, I came up with an answer that I thought I could live with. But that was the point—I was forced to live with myself after bending to the pressure to compromise. I realized then that this would become my life if I allowed myself to become too engaged in electoral politics.

In the end, I gave Dinkins and Koch the same rating. I reasoned that I could not really rate Dinkins higher than Koch, because Dinkins's campaign was just theory at that point; he only had a campaign pledge, and Koch had an actual record. And Koch's record was a pretty good one, if not perfect—and what or who in politics is ever perfect?

We held the press conference on the steps of City Hall to broadcast the results. It was attended by most of the Democratic city politicians. I and a couple of other PCC members held up our choice chart detailing the candidates' ratings for all the world to see: Dinkins, 9.5; Koch, 9.5; Giuliani, 3 . . .

The day after the press conference, newspapers around the region carried an Associated Press report stating that the PCC had hurt Koch's chances in the mayoral campaign since he had tied with Dinkins. Koch, outraged, called the PCC a "pipsqueak fringe group," whining, "Protect me from my friends." This part of politics, the dueling and debating, the responding to attacks, I relished. "I don't think he understands our rating system," I was quoted as saying. "I don't think he understood we rated him in a positive way."

Giuliani had a strong reaction to our ratings, too. I enjoyed watching him trying to twist himself into a pretzel to spin an explanation for his stance that would not immediately position him as anti-choice. After saying he would "uphold the right of choice" and "oppose any attempt to make abortions criminal or illegal" he was called out for flip-flopping on the issue, an accusation that ultimately hurt his campaign.

I MAY HAVE DECIDED not to become a politician or be actively involved in more elections, but I was a trusted figure within the New York City health community. I worked with City Councilman Bob Dryfoos, Senator Schumer, and Comptroller Hevesi—all pro-choice, and all very strong supporters of mine, as I was of them. After the *Associated Press* published a press release of mine urging women to take control of their health, Dryfoos asked me to speak at a town meeting on the topic of monitoring the struggle for women's reproductive rights and to testify in favor of the Women's Health Equity Act of 1990. *Newsday* interviewed me about a bill limiting the testimony defense lawyers were allowed to solicit from crime victims about their sexual past, and I was invited to be part of a panel of respondents to the "Dear Abby" question of the day, "Do we have a responsibility to limit the size of our families?"

I was becoming one of the go-to experts on the feminist point of view, and I commented on an ever-broader range of topics. Some American feminists had a tendency to separate our work on women's equality from other equally important social justice issues, hesitating to speak out on race, class, and global women's rights.[20] I believed that we were all bound by our common potential for victimhood. No matter one's race, one's class, or one's nationality, we were targets simply because we were women. Keeping quiet about an issue for fear of crossing into unknown territory was against the spirit of feminism as I saw it.

In the early nineties New York was plagued by a series of race-related crimes. The media played up the racial aspect of each incident, but they burned in my mind as examples of the sexism that soaked our society. One could not be separated from the other. Yusuf Hawkins, a young black man, was shot dead by police in the white part of town; his death was blamed on Gina Feliciano, a young white woman whose "crime" was daring to break out of her white ethnic ghetto and invite blacks to her home. Another young woman was blamed for her boyfriend's act of setting a fire in a nightclub that killed eighty-seven people. Racism and sexism were present in equal measures in both cases, but the sexism went unreported.

Then came the explosive internationally reported and analyzed Central Park jogger case. From the first reports of the young, white investment banker raped, sodomized, beaten, gagged, and left for dead in Central Park by a group of young black and Latino males, people expressed outrage and astonishment at the randomness and brutality of the attack.

The trial of the five young defendants accused of her rape and attempted murder became a lightning rod for a city already suffering the wounds and anxieties of ongoing racial tensions. The rape was played up to promote paranoia and backlash against men of color. This case was quickly followed by that of Carol Stuart in Boston, who was eventually found to have been murdered by her supposedly well-adjusted, white middle-class husband while pregnant—but only after dozens of black men had been rounded up and wrongly investigated.

In the midst of all the hyperbole and race-baiting, there remained the reality of one young woman whose life had been brutally altered, another who had been murdered, and thousands of others who lived in fear of increasingly horrific sexual violence.

As I wrote in an editorial published in *Amsterdam News*, "Rape is a great equalizer; it has no color and no class." It makes all women sisters, just like unwanted pregnancies do. Indeed, according to trial transcripts, when the Central Park jogger screamed out in pain and panic she was told, "Shut up, bitch." Not white bitch, not black bitch, not rich bitch: just bitch. The same week as the Central Park attack, there were twenty-eight other rapes or attempted rapes in New York City, nearly all of which were ignored by the media. These women were raped, attacked, and murdered simply because they were women.

Sexuality itself, as it was named, defined, sold, and commodified in American culture, diminished women and left them vulnerable to violence. The famous black comedian and political commentator, Dick Gregory, began an address he gave at an Ivy League university by asking his audience, "What do you call a black nuclear physicist?" The answer: "A nigger." It was the same with women. Whatever our race, class, education, age, nationality, and so on, to some people, we were all cunts.

MY PUBLIC PERSONA made Choices a popular target for anti-choice publicity stunts. In June 1990 Brooklyn's Bishop Daily announced to the press that he would lead a prayer vigil outside Choices. "If one is doing the Lord's work, why do you need a press release?" I asked the *Daily News*. He recited the Hail Mary more than 150 times in front of Choices with one thousand demonstrators, but on the day of their protest, none of our scheduled one hundred abortions were canceled.

While Daily gathered his followers to pray on their beads outside my clinic, I was helping to run what I deemed a sort of underground railroad. Women from states with restrictive abortion laws were traveling to New York to have their procedures—just like my first patient who had traveled to my clinic from New Jersey so many years before. I lowered the fees for out-of-state clients and welcomed them to my clinic.

Business was booming. In the early days, when Choices served two to five patients per week, I understood very quickly what women needed from an abortion provider: immediacy of access, affordability, confidentiality, safety, compassion, and dignity. The system I had developed to address all of those needs—creating the ancillary services of the counselors, and leaving the physicians to do the technical work—had proven successful. We grew exponentially until we were seeing over five hundred patients for abortions per week. With my staff of 115 I was basically running a midsize hospital. At our height we performed almost twenty thousand abortions per year, over one hundred per day, making us one of the largest abortion facilities in the United States.

Nearly 97 percent of the abortions were done in the first trimester at a cost of $300. Later term abortions, because of their increased risk, were priced higher. Almost all of the New York clinics charged the same fees. The only price wars were waged by unscrupulous physicians who preyed on illegal immigrant women, charging them unconscionably higher rates, knowing they were afraid to go to a licensed facility for fear of having their status revealed. Abortion, unlike other medical procedures, did not go up in price with inflation. Even so, Choices started to become very profitable. I was quite pleasantly surprised when I made my first million dollars.

I was generous with salaries, including my own and Marty's (who functioned as the medical director), but most of the profits went back into the clinic. I frequently offered new services at Choices and always did my best to subsidize poor women's care. We were famous for never turning a patient away. At least once or twice per week I would get a call from the front desk or a counselor starting with the words, "I have this patient . . ." The power to be able to help them gave me a great deal of pleasure—but I could only have that power if I had the money to service it.

I was the only woman owner of a licensed abortion facility in New York, yet my feminist peers often made me feel as though I was doing something wrong. Many in the movement felt a real activist should be struggling financially, or at least be working for a nonprofit. How, they wondered, could I be a radical feminist *and* a successful entrepreneur? I was "making money off the movement" (which could be said of every abortion provider), even more than most because I was not one of the doctors performing the abortions, but the person who hired them. Male abortion doctors faced less opprobrium, anyway; the fact that they were making money off abortions did not tarnish them the way it tarnished me. I was a woman, a feminist, a radical, a writer, a publisher, and an activist, and I was making a hell of a lot of money. Something wasn't right.

My relationship with money has always been nuanced and complicated. I have felt its deprivation, earned a lot of it, saved it, given it away, risked it, been on the verge of bankruptcy twice, invested it well, and spent it unwisely. I have been envied for it, abused for it, and used for it. Money has given me many types of power. With it I have been able to run my clinic the way I want it to be run, create new programs, and hire talented staff. I have been able to travel and move in worlds I would not otherwise have had the chance to enter.

Money has given me the power to support political campaigns and donate to worthy causes. In the nineties I spent half a million dollars every year publishing *On the Issues* and started a 501(c)3 called the Diana Foundation so that I could donate to feminist groups and individual radicals that had no access to institutional funds.[21] I donated to the campaigns of pro-choice politicians like Schumer and Hevesi, and of course paid for political actions put on by the PCC.

But at times that ability has almost seemed like a one-sided pleasure. It was a brutal education in reality for me to see how so many friends and allies slipped or dropped precipitously away when I almost went bankrupt. Many women were passively resentful of my money. I would go to dinner with friends, and they would apologize for picking a restaurant that was not "one I was used to," although I was as comfortable eating at a diner as I was in an expensive restaurant. It became difficult to know for sure whether people connected to me in true friendship or because of my money. But eventually I came to feel comfortable with this part of my self-presentation. Just as the scandal of my love affair left its residue on me, made me who I am, the distinction of being a wealthy feminist became part of my persona.

IN THE 1980S I noticed an influx of Russian émigrés coming to me for abortion services. The immigration policies of the Soviet Union had eased, and masses of Russians were finding their way to New York City. Abortion was the major form of birth control in the Soviet Union, and many of the women had had ten or twenty before coming to Choices. For these women, the issue of abortion posed no questions of morality, ethics, or women's rights versus fetal life.

I'd been to the Soviet Union once, in 1983, with Marty and a group of his colleagues. A friend who was familiar with the culture begged me to take a suitcase full of contraceptives: pills, diaphragms, condoms. My concerns about arbitrarily distributing hormonal medication and diaphragms that would not be fitted by physicians were laughed off. "They need anything and everything they can get." After learning that the two most popular forms of birth control were douching with lemon juice and jumping on cardboard boxes when periods were late, I stuffed my bags full.

At the time Russia was still a communist country. It was impossible to escape the feelings of state control and oppression. We would get on a bus and no one would smile or meet our gaze; the energy of the place was stifling. I could not stay in a situation where I knew that every word I spoke was being listened to or taped. We left three days early to go to Norway.

The Soviet Union's power to astound confronted me again when a thirty-five-year-old Russian woman came to Choices for her thirty-sixth abortion. The patient expressed relief at the supportive and positive aspects of the clinic as opposed to the brutal conditions with which she was familiar, but seemed quite resigned to having as many abortions as necessary. Like many Russian women, she was violently opposed to using birth control. Most Russian gynecologists promoted the idea that the pill caused cancer, and preached the virtues of repeat abortions. Of course, the fact that many of them subsidized their three-dollar-a-month salaries by doing abortions in women's homes might well have had an influence on their thinking.

The only contraceptive devices locally produced were condoms. These were so poorly made that they were called "galoshes," and few men consented to using them. In Russia the obstetric wards were empty of patients, and one out of three women who sought second trimester abortions in hospitals died from complications. My patients told me story after story of lives blighted by sterility, sexually transmitted diseases, and domestic violence. One woman confided that the brutality of the state maternity wards was Russia's most effective means of family planning. The lack of choice resulted in an alarming number of abortions performed both legally and illegally in Russia. It was impossible to get an accurate number, but it was estimated that between five and 18 million abortions were performed annually as compared to 1.6 million in the United States.

I could not turn away from this situation. In 1992, Joy Silver, the Choices marketing director, arranged for two Russian feminists from *I and We Magazine* who had heard about my facility to visit me. My philosophy of informed medical consumerism astonished them. In Russia, you got whatever treatment was being offered at the moment. If they had a stock of old-fashioned spiral IUDs, that's what was dispensed. If they had high dose estrogen pills, that's what was prescribed, regardless of any individual contraindications or preferences.

When they got home they faxed me an official invitation to lead a team of physicians and counselors from Choices to go to Moscow for an educational exchange. We would be meeting with gynecologists from state-subsidized Teaching Hospital Number 53 to demonstrate state-of-the-art women's health care. Three months later I was on my way to Russia with nine of my staff.

MY HOSTS HAD ARRANGED for us to stay in a prerevolutionary mansion that functioned as a government artist colony where pensioned writers and old artists retired. Marty came along as part of my entourage of Choices staff, a role that infuriated him. He became even more upset when I asked to have my own room; I had a lot of pressure to deal with—giving speeches, meeting international press. I tried to explain this, but Marty perceived it as a public embarrassment in front of the Choices staff, especially the male doctors. Here we were as husband and wife and I was asking for my own room, a public declaration that he did not have sexual access to me. He was sullen and cold, even threatening. "I made you, I can break you," he told me more than once. But I insisted, and we slept in separate rooms.

Resolving to brush off his anger and focus on my mission, I dove into the first day of meetings and interviews. Most of the women I spoke with seemed to be insulated from feminist thought and the feminist movement as we knew it in the United States. They referred to me as Miss or Mrs. Hoffman, and one of my staff corrected them and wrote out "Ms." "But isn't she married?" they asked. I explained that yes, I was married, but that it was not necessary that my marital status be public. They loved that!

There was no word for "counseling" in the Russian system, because they didn't perceive a need for it. Abortion was not only the status quo, but the only choice the majority of women had to control their fertility. There was no organized opposition on religious or moral grounds (although there was a growing American right-to-life presence in Moscow), and women regarded their multiple abortions pragmatically, as a way of "getting cleaned out." I wondered whether bringing to Russia the concepts of choice and responsibility, the need for women to think deeply about birth control and abortion, the need even for counseling prior to abortion, would contribute to an anti-abortion groundswell. Would I inadvertently be introducing anxiety or guilt to an already overburdened and oppressed female population? After all, the slogan of many pro-choice activists in the US—"Abortion on demand and without apology"—was a reality in Russia. But because there were no other choices, abortion had little to do with freedom and privacy and much to do with oppression and coercion.

The day I was to participate in an educational symposium at the Moscow Literary Society, I awoke with an intense feeling of excitement. I would make my presentation and challenge the assembled physicians and journalists to create a truly revolutionary society. During my talk I stressed what I knew to be true in the most personal and political sense: if one accepts that the exercise of free will defines what it is to be moral and fully human, then women who lack the information to make choices are destined to remain second-class citizens.

Along with translated copies of my birth control pamphlet, "Birth Control Facts and Fiction: The Choice Is Yours," T-shirts, and magazines, I had brought seven thousand condoms with me to distribute after the presentations. When the time came to hand them out, the journalists, students, and physicians turned into a swarming mob. I was surrounded as a frenzy of hands reached out to grab the condoms, leaving me breathless and amazed.

My staff was scheduled to perform abortions and Norplant inserts at the state teaching hospital. It would be the first time Norplant had been inserted into Russian women, and the first time abortions would be performed there with state-of-the-art technology. Students, gynecology residents, and the administrative staff of the hospital hovered around the operating room tables. There were three patients in the operating room; multiple abortions were often performed at the same time, without any type of anesthesia. It was faster and more efficient that way. The women came in their own nightgowns because there were shortages of paper supplies. They placed themselves on the table and followed orders.

The next day I had a meeting at the Russian Family Planning Association, one of the only voices calling for a reasoned and intelligent family planning program. The director, Inga Grebesheva, was famous for being the only woman deputy of the Central Committee of the Communist Party. The energy of the women in that room was so strong, I urged them to take immediate action. We decided to draft an open letter to Boris Yeltsin outlining the grave conditions of women's health care and demanding economic funding for birth control and education. I asked Grebesheva if she could have it done by the next day so that leading feminists at the Feminist Roundtable where I would be speaking could sign it. She smiled and told me, "I've been writing it in my head for four years."

When we returned to New York, Marty had a change of heart about the anger he'd felt on our trip. An enormous bouquet of flowers was waiting for me on my desk at Choices on my first day back. The card read, "Darling—you are an international star. With love and admiration, Marty." But I'd already put Marty's dark moods and manipulations out of my mind. I was thinking about Russia.

My trip had received international support, with profiles in the *Economist* and the *London Times* detailing the work I had done there. The Russian media had celebrated my project, proudly displaying my picture on the front page of the *Moscow Times* and reporting that we had "made history" on our trip. Dr. Grebesheva told the press that "until Hoffman suddenly landed on our heads," she had almost given up trying to improve the plight of Russian women. "It is only her enthusiasm and energy that prods me into renewing our own campaign. If Merle wants to start a Choices model clinic in Moscow, we promise to find her premises tomorrow." Indeed,

I was considering replicating Choices there. I could offer Russian women state-of-the-art family planning and counseling, as well as high quality abortion care. Russian women needed a safe harbor, a feminist outpost. I felt I had to do it.

TWO YEARS LATER, with great excitement and a sense of destiny, I boarded the plane for Moscow to build Russia's first feminist medical center. I would call it Choices East. I was aware of the odds: out of thirty-three hundred American/Russian joint ventures formed in 1993 in Moscow, only three hundred were still operative the next year. The American press carried endless stories of the difficulties of doing business in Russia. Apart from the basic challenge of negotiating with people whose core philosophy was for seventy years built around hostility to free markets, I had to take up the challenge of bringing a feminist consciousness to life in a highly misogynist, authoritarian society.

I began thinking in terms of "capitalism with a conscience," a term I coined that had been met with scorn by some American feminists. Perhaps with the enormous economic and political changes in Russia at the time, my take on capitalism would find fertile ground. At that time in Moscow there was what was called soft and hard currency; soft was the ruble, which all the Russians were paid with and used, and hard was the dollar, the franc, the pound, the deutsche mark— the money that was used by foreigners to both purchase goods and bribe officials to get what they needed. I wanted to charge the Russian women for abortions in soft money— about three rubles, equivalent to about fifteen American dollars. I would charge foreign women between $100 and $150 in hard money. The idea was to subsidize the poor women with the profits or surplus that was made from doing abortions on foreigners.

The Russians I spoke with were aghast at this idea. They wanted to have two separate services, one for foreigners and one for Russians—sort of like one for cash and insurance patients and one for Medicaid patients. This surprised me. Wasn't subsidizing the poor a core belief of Communism— "from each according to his ability, to each according to his need"?[22]

Much had changed in Russia since my first exploratory visit in 1992. The rise of fascistic nationalism promoted by Vladimir Zhirinovsky had produced rampant inflation, and growing disillusionment with American capitalism due to the loss of their life savings had left much of the population anxious, frustrated, and despairing. Organized crime had grown at alarming rates, a 43 percent rise in the previous five months. Gang violence, too, was so common that the *Moscow Times* reported a rate of one bomb attack every two days, mainly carried out against bankers and businessmen as gangs battled for control of the city. I'd felt relief on my first visit to Moscow upon discovering that pornography was almost nonexistent, but now I saw it everywhere. The Russian version of *Cosmopolitan* greeted me with the question, "Would you rather have sex or chocolate?" The opening of Russian markets to all things American, like Snickers bars and McDonald's, included imports of our special brands of fundamentalist misogyny: tapes of Jerry Falwell and Jimmy Swaggart now graced Russian television. The American right-to-life movement sponsored a weekly half-hour television program, and a recent right-to-life conference in Moscow boasted five hundred attendees.

I was not surprised to learn that the attacks on me in the press began before I hit the ground. A former KGB general, one Alexander Sterligov, leader of the Russian National Assembly and an ally of Zhirinovsky, was worried that under Yeltsin the mortality rate exceeded the birthrate for the first time since World War II. Calling my plans to set up a women's clinic in Moscow an "anti-Russian ploy," Sterligov was quoted as saying, "We will not put up with Russians having more coffins than cradles." Not only were women the victims of repeat unsafe abortions, now they were being made to feel guilty for having them on both religious and political grounds.

I knew not to graft my American feminist philosophy onto Russian reality. My mission was to work with the Russians on an equal basis; that way they could adapt the Choices philosophy of Patient Power to their Russian sensibilities. The philosophy could then grow organically and be replicated in other parts of the country.

And in this regard things were moving along well. In February I returned to Russia to sign the Protocol of Intent with my partners: the Moscow Clinical Center Marine Hospital and the Department of Marine Transport of the Ministry of Transport. Choices East would be built in the Moscow facility first, and then instituted in eighteen other hospitals.

I took great care in having the legal documents drawn up because the law, like everything else in Russia, seemed to change almost daily. Of particular importance was the division of control. We agreed that both the American and Russian sides would hold equal shares in the venture, sharing in both the potential success and risk of the project. Needless to say, it took many phone calls and faxes to produce the detailed legal documents necessary to form the company.

At the end of my February trip, with much fanfare and press attention, we signed the Protocol of Intent that would lead to our agreement. On my return in the summer, we would finalize and sign the formal documents. Then the real work of setting up the clinic could begin.

In June, my first working day in Moscow was to be spent at the Moscow Clinical Center Marine Hospital. I immediately noticed changes. Our cars were met at the gate by armed guards. The head of the hospital, Dr. Osipov, seemed nervous and distant, his behavior erratic at our meetings. When I questioned my Russian aides about this, they informed me that he had been involved in a business venture that had soured, and had been the victim of an attack that left him in a coma for three months. I began to feel concerned that whatever his motivations, Osipov did not seem willing to move forward on the terms we had agreed upon.

My heart turned cold when he demanded 51 percent of the company. I certainly had never agreed to this. To accomplish anything for women in Russia I needed equal control of the project. Forty-nine percent would render me powerless to control the health care Choices East provided, and would allow my Russian partners to make use of my status, name, and the investments I had arranged. They knew my motivation was not financial gain; the possibility of the clinic making a profit was minimal, and my goal was only to make it self-supporting. I caucused with my aides, who believed that this was a negotiating strategy, political theater designed to gain a controlling share, and that in the end he would sign.

I was on a deadline. I had scheduled a press conference to announce the signing of the agreement; forty international journalists planned to attend. I would have to cancel it. I gave Osipov my ultimatum: by noon the next day he would have to agree to the terms laid out in February, or the deal was off. He looked at me arrogantly and said, "If you are so concerned about saving women's lives, what's one percent to you?"

The next day at noon, I asked Osipov for his decision. His answer, "Fifty-one/forty-nine," hit me like a body blow.

So much work undone, so many hopes dashed. I stood up, shook his hand, wished him well, and walked out of the room. Osipov's aides were amazed. If Osipov was surprised he seemed to hide it well.

The press conference was canceled, but I did give private interviews. The reporter from Izvestia was dismayed. "What will Russian women do now?" she asked me. "How long will they have to wait?" We discussed organizing a grassroots feminist movement. She cautioned me that Russian women would be difficult to mobilize on the issue of women's rights, but that if we could appeal to them to mobilize for the benefit of their children, we would have a better chance. I mused over the irony of women once again reinforcing the traditional role, being there for others and not for themselves. When they tried to be, the results were often fatal. I met with a young American woman who had been working on setting up the first battered women's shelter in Russia. The day she opened the hotline they received four hundred calls. But in the last year, two of the volunteers had been murdered by their husbands.

The visionary in me embraced the pragmatist. I felt disappointed, but not destroyed. I knew I had done the right thing, and that it was not a failure. I had planted seeds in a very dry environment. It was not the right time, but that time would come.

BACK AT CHOICES, I looked into the eyes of the women I served and saw the faces of Russian women, their eyes questioning, hopeful. "How long will women have to wait?"

A conversation I'd had in the hotel leaped into my memory. Svetlana, a dark-eyed Russian journalist, had been writing a newspaper piece about my visit. We were discussing Stalin's criminalization of abortion when she put down her pen and said quietly, "You know, there was some good in what Stalin did. If he had not criminalized abortion, I would not be here."

My mind went to a television debate during which I had been asked, "What would you do if your mother aborted you?" It was the ultimate existential question, the one that plagued so many anti-choice activists, their empathy singularly focused, crushed between self-preservation and hypothetical non-existence.

But there was another hypothetical question to ask: What if Svetlana's mother had had an illegal abortion and perished in the process? That one did not cross her mind. She was giving voice to the assumption that the control of reproduction should be in the hands of the state. She could not see that the State viewed women and their bodies as commodities, property that each state appropriates for its own purpose. They are used as a means of production and a way for the state to exert control over its people.

The comparative history of abortion is actually the history of power relations between states and their female populations. The geopolitical and economic goals of any regime are heavily articulated in its population policy. When Stalin made abortion illegal, allowing Svetlana to be born was not the agenda; the agenda was to populate Russia with soldiers to counteract Hitler's rising militarism. Meanwhile, Aryan women in Nazi Germany who were thought to have aborted their fetuses could be punished with the death penalty, while those deemed "hereditarily ill" were permitted to have abortions.

The battlefields are different, but the war is always the same. For women in sexist, authoritarian societies, the issue of abortion can pose no questions of morality, ethics, or women's rights versus fetal life. There is only the harsh reality that sex rarely comes without anxiety and that the price one often pays for it is high and dangerous.

Romania offered abortion on request until concern over the decline in fertility instigated a change in policy in 1966, severely limiting access to abortion and calling for incentives to childbearing such as birth premiums and tax reductions; the country then legalized them again with the rise of abandoned babies and maternal mortality. Abortion laws enforced by military dictatorships in Chile mandate that women can be jailed for up to five years if they are caught. In China, abortion is considered an important tool for limiting population growth. The legality of abortion in the United States is a wedge issue that flip-flops according to the party in power. And in Russia, women are still being forced to turn to abortion as the primary form of birth control because the state refuses to prioritize their needs.

It is not only the size of population that is subject to control, but the kind; not only the quantity, but the quality. In all of these calculations, women are the losers. True reproductive freedom for women is never under consideration. And so women make the choices they have to make. We navigate the distance and tension between the collectively defined good of society and the good as we individually define it in the context of our own lives. Choice is not a static concept; it expands and contracts depending upon the nature of the regime or the society in which we live.

A Hindu Indian woman, eighteen weeks pregnant, came into Choices with her husband and two young sons, seeking an abortion. She'd had amniocentesis to insure that there were no fetal abnormalities, and found there was nothing wrong with her fetus. Why, then, was she here? What was her reason for wanting this abortion? "It's a girl," she told me. "I can't have a girl. Girls are liabilities."

I thought of the fetus within her and the primal birth defect it carried. I looked at her two sons, holding on to her with unyielding, demanding hands. I felt rage that it was my gender that was the least wanted, and despair over the reality that within this act was a total denigration, denial, and devaluation of the female principle, the female self. I so much wanted to say: "No. STOP! You should not." Not "you cannot," but "you should not."

Yet even as I raged against her choice, I understood why she had to make it. She had left India, but India was where she lived in her heart and her head. Attitudes about abortion are situational, historic, and geographic. The decision to make what in her mind was the only rational and intelligent choice resulted in an ambivalent type of freedom. A freedom that said that in order for a woman to have more than a minimal chance at survival and actualization she must deny and negate her own gender.

But it is for this very fundamental civil right of reproductive freedom that I have put my life on the line many times. Without it, we will never have a world where being female is not considered a birth defect, where women do not have to have thirty-six abortions or be forbidden from having one.

How long will women have to wait?

We will have to wait as long as it takes to bring about women's equality. We will have to wait for people of conscience to create a society where choice truly exists—not one where economic deprivation, racism, sexism, or despair dictates the outcome of pregnancies.

MY THOUGHTS OFTEN turned to philosophy after the experiences I had in Russia. For years, Phyllis Chesler, Letty Cottin Pogrebin, E. M. Broner, and other politically active Jewish women had gathered a group of feminists together for Feminist Seders, during which they took on the roles traditionally assigned to men and retold the ancient tale of Jewish slavery and redemption. The group was growing, and Phyllis invited me to join. When it came to Judaism of any denomination, I always felt a bit removed; most of these women were far more articulate in everything Jewish then I was. I enjoyed being with them, but I always felt like an observer.

But when the Holocaust Museum opened in 1993, I felt myself inexplicably drawn to it. I had been keeping up with the politics, challenges, and questions that had riddled this particular project since its inception over ten years before. How to bridge the distance between memories that remain personalized and mutable, and those which become collectively reified? How to portray the Holocaust as something "outside history" as Elie Wiesel described it, a pathology apart from and outside of any known human parameter but at the same time quintessentially human? In this time of intense secularization coupled with new kinds of spiritual journeys, the Holocaust had become an experience of Jewishness that everyone could relate to.

I had first been introduced to Wiesel as part of my studies in graduate school. His need to tell of the unbelievable evil of the camps, and his burning desire to help prevent the Holocaust's reoccurrence while insuring that the world would not forget its victims drove him to write, and drew me to him. I was transported by his novels and analytic work, which all spoke of his inner journey, his continual search for meaning and god in a world filled with evil and despair. He had a commitment to the moral dimension in life, to the moral answers.

When Mother Teresa, speaking on abortion, said, "We have created a mentality of violence—massive, manipulated, propagandized movements that have brought about more than a million and a half unborn deaths every year," Elie Wiesel didn't agree. The violence he was concerned about was the violence of the abortion debate itself. After reading that he had to think more about abortion and had refused to take a side, I decided that I had to meet with him and discuss it. He agreed to have a dialogue with me for *On the Issues.*

I got off the elevator on the twenty-sixth floor of his New York apartment building, and when I turned left, the first thing I saw was an open door revealing a room with shelves and shelves of books. A small, smiling, intense man waited there for me. I took his hand, met his eyes, and began our conversation.

"When abortion was debated in 1977 in the Knesset in Israel, the anti-abortionists articulated the feeling that abortion was annihilating the Jewish people, that there were no "unwanted" Jewish children, and how can we, after the Holocaust, slaughter Jewish children in the womb? What do you think of this?" I asked him.

"Fanatics are all the same. These are fanatics. I am against fanatics everywhere. I don't understand these words: Abortionist, anti-abortionist. Those who give women the right of choice he or she [sic] is an abortionist? What kind of articulation is that?"

"Yes," I said, "but there is a feeling that women who choose abortions are not active moral agents. That women's reproductive capacities and women's lives are secondary to political ideology or religious morality."

"I don't like generalizations. Some people feel that they need abortion. For them this is their morality. Other people say that for moral reasons they are against abortion. I don't like simplistic definitions."

"You have said that you are uncomfortable with the violence of the abortion debate, but when Cardinal John J.

O'Connor first came to New York, he held a press conference in which he stated that legal abortion was the 'second Holocaust.' How do you feel about abortion being likened to the genocidal slaughter of the Jews?"

"I am uncomfortable with the language of this debate. I resent the violence of the language, the words that they use, like Holocaust—no it is not a Holocaust. It is blasphemy to reduce a tragedy of such monumental proportions to this human tragedy, and abortion is a human tragedy. What should be done is to give back the human proportion to the abortion issue, and when we see it as such we may be able to have much more understanding for the woman who chooses it."

I thought for a moment. "Women who choose abortion are consistently labeled killers, and I personally have been compared to Hitler and called a great murderer."

"A woman who feels she cannot go on, and with pain and despair she decides that she has to give up her child, is this woman a killer?" he mused. "Look, you cannot let these words hurt you. You have to be strong not to pay any attention because those who do that—call you a Hitler and relate it to the Holocaust—prove that they do not know what the Holocaust was."

The Loaded Gun

"If you put a gun on the wall in the first act,
you must use it by the third act."
—ANTON CHEKHOV

Dr. David Gunn was shot three times in the back by pro-lifer Michael Griffin as he was ariving at a Pensacola, Florida, abortion clinic in March of 1993. Griffin yelled, "Don't kill any more babies!" before gunning the doctor down as he stepped out of his car. He was the first provider to be killed in the war against abortion. When I heard that the National Coalition of Abortion Providers was arranging a memorial service in his honor, I knew I had to be there.

Pensacola was enemy territory. There had been a rash of clinic bombings there, and the radical fringe of the anti-abortion movement was particularly active in the area. I was used to living in a war zone, but I was still surprised when Ellie Smeal, president of the Feminist Majority, got on the plane with me and told me that Paul Hill, a notorious anti-abortion activist, had been sighted at the hotel we were to stay in with two unknown aides. An anonymous threat had been made the night before on television by a man whose face was covered by a large, blue dot; we could expect a mass murder, he predicted, something so big that it would surprise both sides, something like Hebron or Beirut. John Burt, one of my old television debating opponents, was quoted on the Pensacola evening news to the effect that he would be getting out of town because the spectacle of two to three hundred abortionists in one place was too much of an incentive for mass murder. He would put himself out of the way of temptation.

Word soon came down that the FBI had intercepted someone in a car loaded with a cache of weapons, headed for the hotel. Agents in Houston had arrested a local antiabortion activist, Daniel Ware, on weapons charges. At his arraignment, evidence was presented to show that Ware had traveled to Pensacola armed with explosives (as well as three guns, one a .357 Magnum, and about five hundred rounds of ammunition) with the stated intention of staging a suicide attack on the abortion providers gathered there.

The morning of the memorial a special meeting was called to discuss defensive strategy. It was agreed that a decision not to go would be respected. Many people were frightened, but no one stayed away. We boarded buses outside our hotel alongside armed police, FBI agents, and members of the Bureau of Alcohol, Tobacco, and Firearms. The reality of driving to a memorial service for a murdered gynecologist in a procession interspersed with motorcycle cops and police cars was one of the more haunting experiences of my life.

The service was held in an amphitheater opposite the clinic. Given the sunny Florida weather, I found it odd that Smeal was wearing a turtleneck sweater with a long, dark blue raincoat. Only after a few minutes of looking at her carefully and noticing that she appeared rather boxy did it occur to me that she was wearing a bulletproof vest. She was not the only one; two male physicians were outfitted with vests, but they were making no secret of it. One walked within twenty feet of a lone picketer holding a sign that read "The wage of sin is death" and "Abortion is murder." As everyone watched, the doctor pounded his chest, screaming, "Why don't you just do it! Come and get me! You don't have the guts." During this display of righteous passion and provocation, Smeal and I stood next to each other scanning the windows that faced the stage, looking for the butts of rifles.

Upon my return to New York, I learned that Rachelle "Shelley" Shannon, an anti-abortion activist, had been convicted of attempted murder in Wichita, Kansas, after she admitted to shooting—though not fatally—Dr. George Tiller, one of the few physicians in the US who specialized in therapeutic late term abortions. Tiller was a friend of mine, and for many years I referred women to his clinic for these difficult procedures. He always wore a bulletproof vest, and drove to work in an armored car. He survived that attack, but he would not be so lucky in 2009.

Two days later, Dr. George Wayne Patterson, owner of four abortion clinics and one of the few physicians to perform abortions in the Mobile/Pensacola area, was killed as he returned to his car in the nightclub district of Mobile. Police attributed his murder to a robbery gone awry, but reports revealed that nothing was stolen from Patterson; his body was left with his wallet on it.

On July 29, 1994, in Pensacola, Florida, the "Reverend" Paul Hill pumped three shotgun blasts into the head of Dr. John Bayard Britton, killing both him and his clinic escort James Barrett and wounding Barrett's wife, June. I had witnessed Paul Hill's crusading in Pensacola during the memorial service for Dr. David Gunn, which he had contaminated with a sign reading "Execute Murderer Abortionists."

Six months later two clinic workers were murdered in Brookline, Massachusetts: Shannon Lowney at Planned Parenthood and Leanne Nichols at Preterm Health Services. Young women doing their jobs—answering phones, copying charts, counseling, teaching, being there for patients—were now seen as collaborators in this abortion "holocaust."

In addition to this sequence of murders, almost two hundred clinics had been bombed since 1977. There had been 347 unlawful clinic entries, 178 death threats, 568 acts of vandalism, and thirty-five burglaries. "Hit lists" of clinic workers circulated among anti-choice organizations. Progressives in the country thought they would be able to rest easy with the election of Bill Clinton, a pro-choice president, but after he took office the war on women went from hot to raging. It seemed that the loss of George H. W. Bush, the antis' friend in the White House, led to feelings of frustration, alienation, anger, and hopelessness—the perfect cocktail to drive some to radical action. Aggressive activism rose in impassioned waves from the anti-abortion movement.

Their madness was also strategic. Anti-abortion leaders knew that without providers, there could be no choice; legal abortion was theoretical if they could frighten doctors away from providing them. Many of the early physicians, whose commitment was formed by the experience of having women die in their arms or in hospital emergency rooms from botched abortions, had died off or were on the verge of retiring. The increasing number of physicians unwilling to perform the procedure because of harassment or lack of commitment and the dearth of medical schools willing to train residents resulted in the need for traveling doctors like David Gunn, who had taken on the burden of providing abortions for multiple counties and sometimes multiple states. The antis' strategy seemed to be working.

As ever, the media's talking heads reassured the public that the murders were random acts of violence, tragedies wrought by psychopathic personalities that had snapped. This placement of the acts within a mental health context had the effect of depoliticizing them. But I viewed this take on the situation as a serious analytic error. The *rhetoric* was the loaded gun; the killers just pulled the triggers. Anyone, emotionally troubled or not, could plug into that anti-abortion message and participate in violent acts fully sanctioned by their peers.

Evidence of the deliberate construction of a climate undermining support for legal abortion and positioning these killers as god's rescuers was ubiquitous. Operation Rescue's Randall Terry, writing in the *New York Post* shortly after the Brookline murders, made it clear enough: "A society cannot expect to tear thirty-five million innocent babies from their mothers' wombs without reaping horrifying consequences. Was it perhaps inevitable that the violent abortion industry should itself reap a portion of what it has so flagrantly and callously sown?" Paul Hill, Dr. Britton's killer, chimed in with an appearance on *Nightline* during which he told the United States that "sometimes you have to use force to stop people from killing innocent children." A Roman Catholic priest, David Trosch, unsuccessfully attempted to place an ad in Alabama's *Mobile Register* that showed a man pointing a gun at a doctor holding a knife over a pregnant woman with a two-word caption: "Justifiable Homicide." Conservative government forces and fundamentalist religious groups were taking advantage of the fact that Americans had no viable external threats on which to focus their attention. They manufactured a very effective abortion narrative that painted providers as the new Soviet threat, an "evil empire,"[23] and offered Americans a new war with which to revive their American manhood.

The antis loved to invoke history—the Civil War, the Holocaust, the Crusades—to add gravitas to their cause, but they were ahistorical at heart. They had crafted themselves into new social beings, "abortion warriors" who existed out of time and space, who engaged in the present with a terrible sense of urgency directing them to act *now*. The pro-choice community took issue with the idea that people could claim to be "pro-life" and support the murder of doctors, but this seemingly contradictive act made perfect sense within the millennialist and apocalyptic zeal of the born-again pro-lifer. Paul Hill and other killers who went to prison were seen as martyrs for the cause.

"I HAVE A GUN. I will be hunting your doctors next week," the voice on the line calmly stated shortly after Dr. Britton's murder in 1994. Choices had been harassed with many bomb threats over its twenty-three years of operation, and I received death threats on a regular basis, but this one was especially frightening.

My staff, which then included seven physicians, was upset and anxious. Although Choices had a group of loyal clinic escorts on duty every Saturday morning to counteract the antis' harassment of patients, they were a meager substitute for twelve-gauge shotguns. My doctors discussed wearing bulletproof vests, but decided against them when they recalled that Dr. Britton had been wearing one when he was shot in the head.

We felt like sitting ducks. I was skeptical of the law enforcement community's will or ability to protect my clinic. It took the murders of three doctors for the government to begin to take anti-abortion violence and harassment against clinic patients and staff seriously. In 1994 the Supreme Court ruled that the Racketeer Influenced and Corrupt Organizations Act (RICO), which was originally intended to be used to prosecute members of the Mafia and other organized crime, could be used against anti-abortion protesters who crossed the line. That same year, President Clinton signed into law the Freedom of Access to Clinic Entrances Act (FACE), making it a federal crime to block access to an abortion clinic or to use force or threats against a clinic's patients. Federal protection was ordered for clinics under siege around the country, and for a moment, greater safety for providers, clinic workers, and patients seemed visible on the horizon.

Then I found out about Henry Felisone and Tony Piso, two New York City residents who had signed Paul Hill's infamous petition describing the use of lethal force in the killing of Dr. David Gunn as "justifiable provided it was carried out for the purpose of defending the lives of unborn children." They lived within a ten-block radius of Choices.

Now was the time to put law enforcement to the test. I called the New York State attorney general to demand protection, and two days later, Washington posted two federal marshals in front of Choices on a twenty-four-hour basis. But the FBI agents who were investigating our threats were new to the intricacies of the FACE act, and I found myself in the strange position of having to coordinate representatives of the civil rights and criminal divisions of the FBI with my local police precinct to begin an investigation of Felisone and Piso on criminal conspiracy charges. I met with the police department's community affairs directors to help educate the cops on the street. When a few weeks passed without further threats, the federal marshals dropped down to guarding Choices for just seven hours a day, and patients came and went as they had for years.

It infuriated me that we had to protect or at least be very involved in protecting ourselves when we were operating a legal, constitutionally protected service. I began a gynecological resident training program at Choices in conjunction with La Guardia Hospital and taught doctors in other facilities

how to search for bombs, the pros and cons of gun owner-
ship, and where to buy bulletproof vests. I called a meeting of
New York abortion providers and representatives of the city's
political establishment to strategize about how to deal with
the escalating violence to clinic patients and staff, and soon
after, convened a summit in Washington, DC, for providers,
pro-choice organizations, and politicians across the country.
The leaders of all the major political lobbying and pro-choice
organizations gathered to discuss the tactics the movement
would need to employ in the coming years.

Wanting to get a sense of what providers experienced in
conservative areas of the US, I sent my activist friend Mary
Lou Greenberg and another member of the PCC to the South
with Refuse and Resist!, a radical human rights activist group,
to learn more about small clinics and doctor's offices that
were particularly vulnerable to attacks. They found that many
abortion providers felt isolated, left to deal with groups of
Operation Rescue members and endless anti-abortion protests on their own. They were ostracized within the medical
community and were often treated as social pariahs. Refuse
and Resist! created a National Day of Appreciation for Abortion Providers (March 10) to support the providers and help
offset their feelings of isolation.

Mainstream leaders of national feminist organizations
urged providers to focus on working with authorities rather
than hiring private security forces and taking matters into
their own hands, for fear of making matters worse by "stooping to the level" of the antis. Some clinic directors were afraid
that counterdemonstrations by pro-choice activists would
give their clinics a circus-like atmosphere. But as Mary Lou
reported, such hesitation was harmful in the long run because
the system could not be relied upon to act in the interests of
women. The PCC and Refuse and Resist! encouraged the clin-

ics to uphold their fundamental right to self-defense against armed attacks—no one else was going to do it for them.

At Choices, I hired more guards and upgraded my alarm and security systems, making every attempt to demonstrate and encourage bravery in the face of this terrorism. We had regular clinic escorts who would courageously come out every Saturday wearing orange Choices vests. I was doing everything I could to keep them safe, but nothing could change the fact that it would take only one act of violence to destroy our fragile sense of security.

Neither was I able to protect my patients from feeling the threat of violence outside the clinic and the anxiety it caused the staff within. They would come in crying and upset after hearing the awful exhortations from the antis' "sidewalk counselors," and indeed, a great part of many counseling sessions was spent dealing with those psychological assaults.

Even though we spoke with every patient individually prior to her abortion, these short sessions were but pebbles in each woman's ocean of need and struggle. There was never enough time to address the shame and fear that so many patients brought to the counseling rooms. It became increasingly clear that abortion could not be extricated from other issues women brought to the clinic—violence at home, abusive relationships, incest, danger on the streets, harassment in the workplace, and economic assaults. It was my daily reality and frustration to see the accompanying despair and hopelessness, the feeling that there was no possibility of change, the feeling each woman had that this was not just her life, but *life*.

As a psychologist I knew something more could be done, as an activist I knew it should be done. I needed to find a way to address each patient's entire experience, body and mind, as a participant in this struggle. One night while I was in bed watching the eleven o'clock news, I saw a piece about how the Mount Sinai Rape Crisis Center, run at the time by Iona Siegel, was going to lose its funding. I sat bolt upright as they interviewed victims of domestic violence who were distraught because they had no other resource. The next day I contacted Segal and met with her about starting a program at Choices.

That moment was the conception of the Choices Mental Health Center. I appointed Mahin Hassibi as the medical director. She supervised the social workers and made herself available to meet the psychiatric, psychological, and spiritual needs of patients and counselors alike. The entire Choices staff, who also deeply felt the pressure of having to absorb the stress of the patients, was eager and willing to participate in the project. They, too, walked past the protesters, and they, too, had to explain to their friends and families that they worked in an abortion clinic. The Mental Health Center would be as helpful to them as it was necessary for the patients.

We knew many women were in abusive relationships but never asked for help. We understood that this reluctance, especially in our large immigrant population, was based on shame and fear of further violence or the potential of breaking up their families. We thought that the most effective way to reach them was through their primary care physicians, the doctors they went to for usual checkups. Many women would go with inchoate complaints—stomach problems, headaches, inability to focus—symptoms of depression that were also symptoms of being a victim of domestic violence. Mahin and I trained the doctors to use a questionnaire we developed to pick up these signs and assess whether the patient needed a referral for mental health treatment, legal services, or both. We developed a new paradigm termed "disorders of intimacy" that allowed us to define domestic violence as a dysfunction of certain intimate relationships. My willingness to see and treat my patients' partners— excluding those who had orders of protection against them, or who were deemed to be immediate threats—led to a great deal of debate on the subject with other feminists involved in the domestic violence community who felt that abusive partners should be immediately removed from the home. But I found that agreeing to work with the partners and employing the concept of "disorders of intimacy" enabled women to feel their own agency instead of inhabiting the role of victim. Our goal was to enable them to be more comfortable asking for help and be more effective at stopping the abuse cycle, and in some cases, preventing the first violent act.

Years before, when I'd worked with the Brooklyn Martial Arts Center, I'd helped teach women how to scream, how to use their voices to resist passivity and the enormous power of the collective conditioning to be "good girls." But as Sally Kempton said, "It's hard to fight an enemy who has outposts in your head." Part of the work of the Mental Health Center was to help women to be present, to feel their power and resist the enemy within and without.

In a sense, the same concept applied to the threatening situation all providers faced. The fact that we were "victims" put us in a kind of female position, waiting for the bully to calm down, hesitating to make too much noise, lest we potentially exacerbate the situation. Like the women who came to us for help with domestic abuse situations, abortion providers and workers collectively held a deep social conditioning that had to be overcome. We had to learn to resist.

ONE EVENING Andrea Dworkin and I discussed the dire situation women in general and abortion providers in particular were facing over dinner at an Afghan restaurant. She said she was questioning the efficacy of nonviolence as a tactic against oppression. With her usual prophetic gravitas she told me she had begun to think about using force, of fighting back against those who would take our lives in their hands.

I was not surprised to hear this. The zeitgeist was definitely changing; there was a palpable, inescapable sense of resistance in the air. When *Thelma and Louise* hit the theaters, women saw themselves in the two friends who transgressed every barrier and protected each other to the death. Women identified with the characters' sense of personalized justice rather than lawfully bound definitions of right and wrong. You rape me or my friend, I kill you. You mess with my freedom, I leave you. And, ultimately, you try to kill me, I kill myself, because death is superior to your laws around me.

I thought of the antis marching in front of my clinic, threatening my staff with bombs, seemingly unstoppable forces who believed they were doing god's work. It was maddening to be unarmed, defenseless, while the antis openly spoke of murdering our forces, then acted on their word. We activists had all been taught that pacifism was generically feminist, that gains could be made through patience and careful, legal steps forward. Yet for every woman served by Choices and Choices Mental Health Center, unknown numbers were suffering violence. I could hold summits, teach my staff self-defense, and publish dozens of editorials in *On the Issues*, but, as Elie Wiesel said, "One man with a machine gun can kill a thousand sages."

I knew that things had changed when I was handed a button that read "I'm Pro-Choice and I shoot back" at an abortion providers conference in Washington, DC. Six years before, when the danger had involved only invasions, harassment, and bombings, the buttons and bumper stickers read "I'm Pro-Choice and I vote."

Doctors hadn't signed up for this. When they first began to perform abortions they were viewed as progressives, or mavericks. Now they were living in a constant state of post-traumatic stress. Any attack on another provider struck fear and terror in them, which is exactly what the antis wanted. One physician in Nevada had built a million-dollar clinic outfitted with strategic military defense protection and six .357 magnums. He called it Fort Abortion. The late Dr. William Harrison of Arkansas bravely announced, "I have chosen to ride this tiger unquietly, raking its side with verbal spurs, swinging my hat and whooping like a cowboy." No matter how they chose to handle their plight, doctors had been forced to join the battle.

The gun was on the wall; were we nearing the right time to use it? In order to minimize my vulnerability, I purchased a twenty-gauge, pump-action Mossberg shotgun at a small shop on Garrison's Main Street to keep at home for self-protection. I shot at tin cans in the woods behind my home to practice my aim, and before long my neighbor noticed the noise and called the police. A *Daily News* journalist got wind of my purchase from the police blotter and wrote under the headline "Make Her Day": "If you've noticed the Right-to-Life crowds thinning in front of Choices Women's Medical Center in Queens, maybe it's because the abortion clinic's president, Merle Hoffman, just purchased a shotgun." There was a negative reaction from some of my feminist colleagues, especially my *On the Issues* editor Beverly Lowy, who was aghast. "Gloria Steinem will be very upset," she told me. A feminist with a gun? It was politically incorrect.

THE RELENTLESS PRESSURE was compounded by the first patient death at Choices, a thirty-six-year-old Haitian woman who died of an amniotic embolism, a rare but almost always fatal phenomenon that is unforeseeable and unpreventable. Her name was Alerte Desanges.

Even though everything that could have been done to save her had been done, and even though there was no way to prevent or to identify the possibility of the event even occurring, I had a tremendously difficult time with this fatality.

I took many trail rides on Hollywould, my beautiful Arabian horse, trying to come to terms with the reality of her death—and the challenge of having my face and Choices smeared all over television, radio, and print media. These catastophic events happened everywhere, but this one happened at Choices, and that made all the difference. I was forced to make an excuse for something that was impossible to make an excuse for. Since I was not a medical doctor, I was dependent on my physicians' expertise—but as the CEO of Choices, I was ultimately responsible for what happened there.

Dr. David Gluck, who had performed the abortion, had previously had his license suspended because he'd been writing illegal prescriptions to fund his gambling habit. He was an excellent doctor, though, and an ally wholly committed to women's reproductive freedom. Marty's recognition of this and his willingness to hire and supervise Dr. Gluck at Choices during the five years of his probation had saved his career. Now, his past indiscretions complicated the otherwise straightforward incident of Desanges's death, giving the press the chance to question the medical standards at Choices and our employment of Dr. Gluck.

I told reporters that it was in the American character to give people a chance at redemption, hoping that word might strike a chord. But the media was hungry for stories about abortions gone wrong, ready to cast abortion doctors— never referred to as physicians—as the pariahs of medicine.

Well-run, safe clinics like Choices were lumped together with "bargain butchers" who took advantage of poor women or undocumented immigrants who felt they couldn't turn to a licensed facility for services. When the trial of Abu Hayat, the "Butcher of Avenue A" who botched the abortion of an eight-month-old fetus, leaving the woman hemorrhaging and her daughter with only one arm, hit the press, anti-choice groups used the opportunity to call again for a law declaring the fetus a person with constitutional rights. The pro-choice movement stayed quiet on the issue, hesitating to comment lest they dig themselves even deeper into the hole the press had put them in. We could not defend Hayat—what he did was unconscionable—but we had to make it clear that safe providers existed, too. The department of health was largely responsible for the hypocrisy and politicization of the issue; licensed facilities were held to extremely rigid standards, yet unlicensed facilities were not held to task when they "illegally" (according to a New York State law that was never enforced) performed second trimester abortions, leading to dangerous situations in which doctors were performing twenty-four-week abortions in their own offices.

WELL-PUBLICIZED botched abortions brought second- and late-term abortion procedures, which are more physically and psychologically trying for both patients and doctors than first-term procedures, under public scrutiny. Indeed, when Choices had gone "up" in gestation in the mid-eighties by offering second-term abortions, even I found the process to be emotionally difficult. The results of choice were not diffused and amorphous, but observable and definable.

The only second-trimester procedure offered at the time was the saline abortion, in which saline was injected into the uterine cavity to kill the fetus, after which labor was induced.

Due to medical considerations, saline abortions could not be performed until the woman was sixteen or seventeen weeks pregnant. Aside from the fact that a woman who was twelve weeks pregnant (the cut off for first trimester abortions) had to go through the trauma of waiting five weeks to have an abortion, when she entered the hospital to expel the fetus she faced another special kind of hell: abortion patients were placed in the maternity ward of the hospital next to mothers who were giving birth, and many became the targets of anti-abortion sentiments.

Wanting their patients to avoid that experience, gynecologists eventually developed dilation and evacuation (D and E), a technique where the fetus was dismembered within the woman's uterus and removed. D and E's were much safer and psychologically easier on the patient since they could be performed at any point after twelve weeks and did not require the woman to go through a delivery. But the procedure was difficult for the doctor and staff performing it—and difficult for the public to stomach. As debates about fetal pain entered the public discussion, some physicians began routinely injecting and killing the fetus with digoxin prior to the abortion itself, eliminating the possibility that the fetus might experience pain.

Graphic descriptions of the procedure, as well as misconceptions about how and why it was performed, added to the stigmatization of providers. These late-term procedures were done only under rare circumstances in which the mother's life or health were at risk or it was determined to be a safer procedure by the physician. But antis focused on the difficult, traumatic procedure itself rather than on the fact that it was only performed when medically necessary. Learning that in some critical late-term cases the fetus was partially dismembered, and the skull crushed, outside the birth canal—a procedure called intact dilation and extraction (IDE)—antis renamed the procedure "partial birth abortion," using physiological geography to further advance their claim that the procedure was no different from murder.

The 1996 case of Amy Grossberg and Brian C. Peterson, Jr., two high school sweethearts charged with intentionally killing their newborn son and abandoning him in a dumpster, was publicly twisted by the antis into a parable with a pro-life moral. Arguing that the Peterson-Grossberg neonaticide was merely an extension of a late-term abortion was a particularly insidious style of political spin, similar to the arguments that fetuses were analogous to Jews during the Holocaust or blacks during slavery. And like "aboritoriums," "abortion mills," and "Hitlers," "partial birth abortions" became a hot-button term used to manipulate the truth about the hows and whys of abortion in the eyes of the public.

Ron Fitzsimmons, the founding executive director of the National Coalition of Abortion Providers (NCAP), publicly said that he'd lied in 1995 when he told Ted Koppel on *Nightline* that there were only five hundred "partial birth abortions" in the United States each year, stating the number was actually over five thousand. He implied that all abortion providers had agreed to be deliberately dishonest about how often IDEs were performed on patients. As Frank Rich wrote in the *New York Times*, Fitzsimmons was not himself a provider, he was a lobbyist, and the "shocking" revelation of the number of IDEs performed each year was already common knowledge. But the damage had been done, and anti-abortion activists reacted with glee, publicizing Fitzsimmons's lie as if they'd uncovered a conspiracy.

I was furious. He was a hired gun who had shot himself and the pro-choice movement in the foot, and I didn't want him to get away with it. NCAP had played a very important role for providers since its inception in 1990 and I had worked closely with them to develop their organizational philosophy. It was a coalition of smaller, independent providers that acted as a balance to NAF, which was heavily loaded with Planned Parenthood leaders and interests. Planned Parenthood was quite different from the smaller facilities and clinics, and it had access to political power and money for nonprofit activities that allowed it to become a fierce competitor of smaller, but equally important, doctors' offices and abortion clinics. Fitzsimmons had sabotaged the reputation of a very important vehicle for women's choice. The reaction of many of the women of NCAP mirrored the "stand by your man" persona of political wives who supported their philandering or criminally involved husbands. But I pulled out of the organization, recalling a $10,000 grant I had given them. I thought he should have fallen on his sword, at least—and if he wouldn't, someone else should have helped him to do it.

Perhaps the worst effect of Fitzimmons's debacle was its political impact. Some pro-choice leaders were willing to publicly oppose IDEs as a way to appease the antis. After a *New York Times* article on the issue broke, the House revisited and approved the Partial Birth Abortion Ban Act by an even larger veto-proof majority than it had the previous year. It gave some normally pro-choice, progressive Democratic senators reason to vote for legislation that placed women's right to choose in increasing jeopardy.

The antis had found a way to incorporate their agenda into the democratic platform, and they were being given free openings. More pro-life Democrats began demanding equal access to the Democratic platform and powerful committee positions, and in the name of the "big tent," the Democrats handed it over. They nominated Dr. Henry Foster, Jr., a moderate physician who publicly stated that he "abhorred abortion," for the position of surgeon general, and even invited Harold Ford, Jr., an anti-choice House representative from Tennessee, to give the keynote speech at the 2000 Democratic National Convention.

The antis had effectively transcended the bifurcation of the Right and Left on the issue of abortion. Combining the "right to life" with other progressive causes, antis could find a home wherever they were on the political spectrum. Many people who described themselves as politically pro-choice began to feel the need to say, "I don't like abortion, but . . ." while political leaders regularly followed President Clinton's adage that abortion should be "safe, legal, and rare."

As a pro-choice president Clinton did deserve credit for his two vetoes of the "partial birth" abortion bills, but his willingness to cater to the Blue Dog Democrats, and increasingly the Republicans, was becoming a political problem. At the UN Population and Development Conference in Cairo Vice President Al Gore, bending to pressure from the Catholic Church and its fundamentalist allies, assured the attendees at the conference that "the United States has not sought, does not seek, and will not seek an international right to abortion." He cemented the US government's position that reproductive freedom was not a transcendent human or civil right, but merely a local privilege that could be granted, limited, or denied according to national customs and laws. This may have been situational diplomatic maneuvering, but it read as gender-specific noblesse oblige.

And then there were the turncoats. The pro-choice movement had always had defectors—people like Dr. Bernard Nathanson (the owner and operator of CRASH, one of the nation's first and largest abortion clinics, who went on to produce the anti-choice film classic *The Silent Scream*) who had a public change of mind and heart. Thanks to Clinton and Gore the numbers began to increase at an alarming pace. Norma McCorvey,[24] a.k.a. Jane Roe, the original poster girl for choice, was the most famous example of this particular social and political trend. It has always amused me that people can find Jesus in the strangest of places; when news broke that McCorvey had gotten herself baptized in a Texas swimming pool by a leader of Operation Rescue, I was not surprised. Reverend Flip Benham, who did the honors, reported that Jesus Christ "had reached through the abortion mill wall and touched the heart of Norma McCorvey." "I've cheated people out of money," McCorvey told Ted Koppel in a *Nightline* interview on August 15. "I've sold drugs. I've done a lot against his teaching. But I think the greatest sin that I did was to be the plaintiff in *Roe v. Wade.*"

Feminist Naomi Wolf argued in *The New Republic* that the pro-choice movement had committed three mortal sins: "hardness of heart, lying, and political failure." She posited that by using the language of communitarianism, positioning abortion rights within a paradigm of traditional Judeo-Christian rights and responsibilities, the pro-choice movement would be able to expand its political base to include the all-encompassing middle where most Americans felt comfortable. To my thinking, this strategy would only operate as a Trojan horse to bring the enemy's arguments into the heart of pro-choice territory, potentially tearing the movement apart.

Wolf concluded her piece by calling for a fantasy of a world where "passionate feminists might hold candlelight vigils at abortion clinics, standing shoulder to shoulder with the doctors who work there, commemorating and saying goodbye to the dead" (the unborn, the never to be born). In the real world I lived in, passionate feminists were desperately needed to stand shoulder to shoulder with doctors and clinic workers to help protect them against the Michael Griffins, Paul Hills, and John Salvis who shot them down in cold blood. We were facing expansions of the Hyde amendment, increased clinic violence, limits on federal employee health insurance, denial of abortions to women in the military, and the reinstatement of the global gag rule. Where was her anger? Where were Thelma and Louise? I didn't care about the rhetoric and rituals of memorials and lighting candles for the dead. I wanted the sisterhood to light the fires of resistance in the living.

That spirit of resistance had already begun to fade, replaced by politically institutionalized actions. The anti-choice and pro-choice movements were operating as sophisticated political campaigns, using visuals, metaphors, debating points, and strategies to construct abortion narratives that would win over the masses. The media contributed by perpetuating the kind of soulless sports mentality that registered everything in neatly competitive categories: Right-to-life 2, Pro-choice 0. Cable channel New York 1 even wanted me to debate two right-to-lifers on the issue of whether or not murdering doctors was justifiable homicide. I declined. The fact that this debate was even proposed was indicative of the backslide the movement had undergone.

The words "pro-choice" were no longer descriptive of the women's movement on anything but a theoretical, ideological level. People felt it was necessary for the movement to cloak and soften the crushing reality of abortion in order to instill in people the knowledge that it was absolutely necessary for women's survival and participation as full citizens in this society. But women's rights, women's lives, and women's equality and autonomy wouldn't sell in the American marketplace, no matter how appealingly they were presented. In the struggle to win the hearts and minds of the American people, the pro-choice and women's movements had to take care not to lose their souls.

IN A CHANGING political climate in which even the Left could not be counted on to support abortion clinics and providers, it was more important than ever for me to keep Choices functioning at its highest level. The women who came to us seeking abortions did not care about Bill Clinton's flip-flopping or communitarianism. They just needed abortions.

I always had to make tough choices to ensure their needs were met, but in the mid to late nineties, gut-wrenching decisions seemed to be part of my daily fare. I had been subsidizing my Mental Health Center with the surplus revenues of Choices to keep it alive while working to get it licensed, after which I assumed it would support itself. But mental health patients were always the stepchildren of the health care system. Insurance and Medicaid rates were not high enough to pay providers, and limits on the number of mental health-related visits made it hard for patients to get the care they needed. Subsidizing these expenses drained Choices, contributing to an extreme cash deficit.

The situation was compounded further by an avalanche of economic and political attacks. Choices' twenty-year lease was up, and it was time to negotiate a new one. But my landlord, Sam LeFrak, had ceded the management of his real estate corporation to his son Richard, who had very different politics from his father. When it came within one year of discussing the possibility of signing another lease, Richard LeFrak made it clear to me that he had no intention of having an "abortion center" continue to be a tenant in his building. If I was not out by the end of the lease, he told me, I would be forcibly evicted.

He had already signed a contract with CompUSA to take over my lease at the end of a three-month holdover period, and he threatened to "bulldoze" my space if I remained one extra day. But it was nearly impossible to find a new building and move the entire clinic with so little warning. We petitioned the court to keep our doors open until we could get a new space ready, and dozens of letters of support were sent by prominent members of the community to the civil court of Queens County in 1998. "This is more than a landlord/tenant dispute—this action threatens to impact the health and safety of many Queens County residents," wrote Geraldine Ferraro. Yet the courts ruled against me, and I was forced to liquidate my entire savings to cover the costs of speeding up the construction of the new site.

When we finally did move into our new space (at which time it was only 70 percent finished) in October of 1997, we found that we'd simply gone from one crisis to another. Six months after I had signed the lease, the building had been sold to an owner who was anti-abortion—and committed to making my life miserable. Tim Ziss, the owner's representative, attempted by any means possible to prevent me from moving into the new space, trying to make me change the layout from the front door to the back of the building—in essence, attempting to change our address. When I refused, Ziss did not allow the contractors to work, again jeopardizing the operation. The extent of the harassment was so severe that I had to call Attorney General Janet Reno's office, which provided armed federal marshals to guard my space during the last few months of construction.

Over the next two years, Ziss left Choices without heat or air conditioning, and unfinished roof work resulted in multiple floods. All of these financial pressures forced me to delay paychecks, forgo my salary for six months, purchase supplies on personal credit cards, implement pay cuts, lay off staff, and suspend all advertising, resulting in a drastic reduction in my patient population.

Then came the ultimate test: should I choose theory or practice, vision or pragmatism, ethics or survival? I had only enough money to either meet payroll and get supplies, or to pay taxes. Opting to survive, I accepted the fact that I would have to deal with my tax situation when it arose, hopefully far in the future. I stopped paying them—the point was to have a future.

By now I was living on pure adrenaline, going from one lawyer to another as I tried to stave off bankruptcy, keep the builders working, the clinic open, the patients safe, and my own sanity intact. Just as with the indictment, Marty was having difficulty keeping himself psychologically together. He often told me he felt weak, and he had difficulty walking long distances. He was nearly eighty years old.

I REMEMBER EMBRACING Marty in the hallway outside of my studio apartment in Queens in the full flush of passion, telling him that I would love him forever, that things would never change between us. He looked at me with a poignancy that struck me as strangely sweet at the time. "No," he said, "I will age, and it won't be the same." And he was right. In a brutally honest, yet gentle discussion, we acknowledged we were no longer meeting each other's needs. We still loved each other, but we knew we had to let each other go. He began to spend his weekends in Florida while I stayed in Garrison. We were not legally separated, but we arranged to have split custody of the house.

Despite all that, we were still allies. When Marty turned eighty, I wanted to honor him, our marriage, and our partnership. He was never really recognized by the powers at HIP for all his important work, and I wanted to give him the retirement dinner they never had for him. I threw him an eightieth birthday party at the Tavern on the Green in Central Park and invited many of the HIP colleagues and personal friends of his who were no longer friends of mine.

About a month before he died we had dinner at one of our old favorite Italian restaurants in Greenwich Village. Having recently spent so much time apart, we began to reflect on our relationship. We expressed how much we had given one another, and how sorry we were for the hurt we had caused each other just by being ourselves.

I arrived home at my apartment late one Sunday evening after an event. When I flipped on my answering machine I was greeted by my sister-in-law's voice. "Merle, Merle, it's Marty. He had a heart attack. He's gone." Click.

I erased the message and sat in silence. After what seemed an immeasurable amount of time, I picked up a pen and spent the night writing Marty's obituary.[25]

BY THE TIME of Marty's death I had come to know myself enough to be able to apologize to his ex-wife, Bernice, at the funeral, for all the pain I had caused her. Indeed, with Marty's death, my eviction, and the constant stress of being a pariah, I thought I knew everything there was to know. But there was another lesson in reality waiting for me. I had never really felt that the world had lost its moorings, never questioned the certainty of my own survival, until I was betrayed, soon after Marty's death, by one of my doctors, Alan Zarkin. He brought me the closest I had ever come to my own destruction. He was the worst of my paid enemies.

Marty had taken Zarkin on as another of his pet projects, "rescuing" him after he came under fire for a drug addiction problem—all too common with doctors in high stress fields. I'd worked with him off and on for years, and I knew him to be an excellent physician, someone who had struggled with his addiction demons and triumphed, and a good Jewish son who took care of his mother. But one day I received a complaint from a lawyer naming Zarkin as the plaintiff. This in and of itself was not very unusual; a busy medical center receives complaints, requests for charts, and other legal documents on a fairly regular basis. I read through it quickly until my eyes came upon the words "carved two inches high into her stomach." I went back and read it again, transfixed. Zarkin was being accused of carving his initials into a patient's stomach after he delivered her baby at Beth Israel Hospital, where he had worked before coming to Choices. I picked up my phone and paged Zarkin, who was on the second floor doing cases.

When he entered my office I waved the legal papers in his face. "Is this true?" Without even asking me what the papers were, he answered calmly, "Yes."

I had the sickening feeling inside my stomach that one gets when falling off a very high cliff in a nightmare.

I called my management team and my lawyers for an immediate meeting in my office, during which it was revealed that Zarkin had been sued for this carving in the past and had lied to me on his medical application when asked whether he was accredited to work at Beth Israel. He was not. I was sitting in amazed silence, still shocked, when Zarkin announced, "If you have nothing else for me to do I have to catch a plane for Paris." I told him he was fired.

The first phone call came from the *Daily News*, and then the games began. Dr. Elahi, the medical director I had hired Zarkin to replace because of his incompetence, told the *New York Times* he thought I'd known about Zarkin's act when I hired him—a lie. But Dr. Elahi had known, my administrator had known, and Beth Israel had known, and they had all neglected to inform me that I had hired a compromised physician. The Department of Health had known, too, but since they were required to give Zarkin "due process," they kept me in the dark, letting Choices take the fall.

I was familiar with the manipulation of the media, acutely aware of how one word, one turn of phrase, could create new worlds. New headlines greeted me each morning. The *Queens Courier*: "Clinic Director Says, 'Dr. Zorro Betrayed Me.'" The *New York Post*: "Abort-Clinic Deaths Didn't Nix His Career"; "Probed Doctors Aren't Feeling Much Pain"; "Mark of Zorro Remains a blight on NY Women"; "Zorro Clinic should be out of abortion biz"; "Zorro cut some slack." And the *Tablet*: "Abortion Is a Dirty Risky Business." I tried to protect myself when I gave an interview to the *New York Times* by having my lawyer on the other end of the conversation, but the piece was essentially a smear job, and my reputation in the field, which had been the best in the industry, was blasted to pieces.

Newspapers called ex-employees who were living in other states to try and pull up dirt about me. Reporters pushed their way into Choices, and someone sneaked in with a hidden camera posing as a patient to see if they could find anything. Confidential files were stolen from my office. Memos that I had written were flashed across the screen on prime time. My enemies watched and waited. People who were very close to me, people who were working for me, competitors, feminists, politicians—everyone was quick to believe what they read about me and the clinic. Even the women with whom I had fought on the barricades, people I had mentored and trained in radical abortion politics, were not there to support or defend me.

The next lie told by the *New York Times* hit Choices harder than anything that had come before: "Queens Clinic being investigated for Medicaid Fraud." This was patently untrue. I was undergoing a routine audit like all other regulated health care providers, and if they found anything that they perceived as suspicious it would be referred to the attorney general. No issues were found, but the consistent negative publicity led to the loss of many longterm referral sources, an inability to recruit new staff, and ultimately, the near bankruptcy of the clinic.

It also left an opening for the Department of Health to go after the clinic with a vengeance. Antonia Novello, the health commissioner at the time who was later indicted for having abused her power during her seven-year tenure, had a personal anti-choice agenda. During a speech she made to a pro-choice group, she announced that she intended to go "hunting bear" at Choices the next day, looking for anything she could find to shut me down. Novello subsequently published a negative report detailing Choices' infractions: our medical records were not organized according to the DOH's specifications, the doctors' signatures were not always legible, and we had difficulty with heating the facility due to problems with the landlord. She had gone searching for problems to make a political point. Choices was given a $60,000 fine, $40,000 higher than that of Beth Israel, where Zarkin had actually done his dirty work. I was ordered to close the clinic for two weeks, while Beth Israel was allowed to continue to operate without interruption. Their only casualty was Dr. Daniel Saltzman, the head of the OB/GYN department of Beth Israel at the time, who had known about Zarkin's act when he came to Choices for a meeting to institute a referral agreement for prenatal patients with him. Saltzman had been fired by Beth Israel shortly after that meeting.

The DOH sent their operatives into the clinic the morning after Novello shut us down and put their fingers in the sinks to check whether we had used them in the middle of the night. It reminded me of Marty's description of the Midnight Express—abortion by candlelight.

In a way, the patients had a better sense of reality than the media or the movement. Even when we were closed, they continued to show up for services. The Department of Health had developed a list of places to which the abortion patients—about 250 a week at the time—could be referred, but amazingly, some of these "facilities" were unlicensed doctor's offices that didn't even have anesthesiologists. The Department of Health wasn't living up to its own standards. The patients preferred to follow my recommendations instead, trusting my judgment. Every morning when they arrived they willingly boarded buses I hired to take them to the Brooklyn Ambulatory Surgery Center, a licensed clinic that arranged to accommodate our patients in their facility.

After the two weeks were finally up and Choices had answered all the numerous citations of the Department of Health, I was told that I could begin to treat patients again. I was relieved, excited to get back to work and serve those who had loyally come back to Choices. There were about sixty patients in the waiting room the morning we reopened. My lawyer came into my office with a strange look—and more bad news. Ziss had reported to the Department of Buildings that I had been operating in his building for years without an appropriate certificate of occupancy. This was entirely untrue—I could never have opened in that location in the first place without Department of Buildings approval—but nevertheless, the claim had to be investigated. We were forced to close for one more week.

The Zarkin scandal had metastasized into losing long-standing referral sources, competitors taking advantage by feeding negative publicity, patients believing that Choices was closed for good, staff leaving because the press was harassing them at home, and international defamation of Choices and myself. To this day people come up to me and ask, "Does that crazy doctor still work for you?"

I HAD BEEN instrumental in defining the reality that it was not politics, but necessity which brought women to choose abortion. The only thing that bound them together, the primal commonality, was the physicality of the thing itself. The legs spread apart, the speculum, the suction machine—that never changed. But everything else had become a mediated reality. I wanted to go back to the beginning, when there was just me and my consciousness, not even informed by feminism. I longed for true solitude.

I stopped debating and giving speeches. In 1999 I suspended publication of *On the Issues*. The bomb threats, Marty's death, the eviction from a space I had leased for twenty years, and my inability to subsidize the magazine anymore overcame my need for artistic expression. Looking back, I see now that I was in a constant state of agitated depression. Abortion had become as codified politically and institutionally as anything else. It was exhausting.

The adventures I had with Mahin were the only respite for me during these times. She understood my internal struggles more than anyone else, and I could be totally myself with her. On the eve of my fiftieth birthday we found ourselves in an old Russian helicopter, rising thousands of miles over the Himalayas. To further remove myself from materiality, I went to Nepal, a world that was, ironically, intensely physical. From Everest, where the rarefied atmosphere creates a constant focus on one's breath, to Katmandu, where the fog of pollution and the stench of poverty and incense do the same, I found myself aware of my senses, surrounded by an endless cycle of death, birth, and rebirth that triggered a rush of physical memories of my own history.

What did being fifty mean for a woman?

I thought of the last twenty-five years: building Choices, defining and realizing a world where women's lives and women's realities were named and validated; the thousands of women who came expecting and receiving safety, compassion, and understanding; all the lives I touched, all the lives that touched mine; my deferred dream of doing the same for Russian women; all the great and small political battles fought and those still to come. Worlds away from Choices, I remembered the seeds of my passion.

I kept moving. I flew to South Africa to work with a rape crisis center. I traveled to Iran with Mahin, entering her country curiously, and somewhat apprehensively. In a sense, Iran entered me. Dressing as a Muslim woman in a chador, I moved awkwardly into a socially constructed invisibility. But remarkably, by the time I left Iran I would find the restrictive coverings an unexpected revelation. I felt totally concealed, yet strangely naked at the same time. Free from an individuality defined by attire, and with only one's face exposed, the presented "self" became more focused and authentic. For the first time, I inhabited a space without familiar roles or stereotypic assumptions.

I traveled alone to the Galápagos. I experienced the barren, dry black lava with a breathless expanse of twilight-blue sky. At night there were so many stars I was able to lose myself in the sky, to reflect. I thought about my new life without Marty. At first I had struggled with my aloneness, with not having someone there to *leave* me alone. I had maintained the questionable belief that a romantic partnership could fill some void or truly fulfill me. Soon, though, I found that I no longer believed that. I knew how to fill myself.

Amazing Grace

"I was going to die, if not sooner then later,
whether or not I had ever spoken myself. My silences had
not protected me. Your silence will not protect you."
—AUDRE LORDE

Welcome to my world." My words were published in the *New York Post* on October 17, 2001, just a little over a month after the 9/11 terrorist attack on the World Trade Center. It was a controversial statement, but it was the truth. Envelopes filled with anthrax were sent to television stations and five US senators instigated national panic, but I was used to checking my mail for white powder every day. Grand Central Station was threatened with a bomb, but I'd been looking under my car for signs of foul play, my heart beating quickly in anticipation of an explosion, for a decade by then. I'd been avoiding windows for fear of bullets since Barnett Slepian was gunned down at his kitchen window in front of his wife and children in 1998. I tensed my body every time I walked from my car to Choices.

When a friend called me the morning of 9/11, telling me to turn on the television, I felt not shock, but powerful despair as I watched the second plane hit. I called Choices, told my staff to send the patients home, got dressed, and drove over the Fifty-Ninth Street Bridge. There, on that perfect fall day, I could see the black smoke rising in the background to my right. At the clinic, my staff and I hovered around the radio and waited for directives until it became clear that I should evacuate the building. We hurried outside together, promising to keep in touch. I stepped into my car and turned on the radio just as it was announced that New York was under a terrorist attack, and people should not be driving in the city. Fortunately it was still early, so I was able to cross the bridge back into Manhattan.

Two days later, a friend and I drove down to the site of the attack. We parked some blocks away due to the phalanx of police protection that prevented us from coming within a mile of the site. I could smell the charred remains of the towers and see the black, dripping steel rising high from the smoldering ground. Already the hawkers with their souvenirs camped out on the sidewalks. Looking into the dazed faces around me, I sensed that we all shared the same reality. In the stores, on the trains, on the streets, everyone had a sense of connectedness that I had never experienced before. We were in a war zone and we had no idea what might be coming next. The immediate shock and fear of another attack was slowly replaced by searing grief, anger, and rage.

New York State attempted to provide mental health support to those affected by the attack through a program called Project Liberty, a collaboration between the Office of Mental Health, local governments, and nearly two hundred local agencies that provided free and anonymous mental health services throughout the declared disaster area. Choices, like other mental health centers, wanted to do what we could, so we offered immediate and long-term services through the program. For many, the physical wound on ground zero was a smoldering metaphor for emotional and psychological wounds that would never heal.

"How could this have happened?" I never asked that question. My body and mind were used to living in a constant state of functional anxiety, and as I absorbed this blow like the others that had come before, I wondered at myself for not reacting with more emotion.

THE ATTACKS OF 9/11 provided an ideal context for Bush to lead his holy crusade as the god-ordained protector of American citizens, born and unborn. All Americans were awash in a sea of righteous patriotism. This was not the time for questioning or opposition to a "war president." It was the perfect environment for Bush to attempt to fulfill his campaign promise to enact a deeply conservative reproductive and sexual agenda with the ultimate goal of banning abortion.

On January 22, 2001, the twenty-eighth anniversary of *Roe v. Wade* and President George W. Bush's first full day in office, he reinstated the draconian "gag" rule, restricting funding for international family planning and denying medical information on abortion to poor women treated at federally funded clinics. The Bush administration's opening salvo made it perfectly clear that the US was going to use its enormous power and prestige to tell the world in no uncertain terms that girls' and women's lives were not important.

In the wake of 9/11, Bush followed his first act as president by withholding $34 million in funding for women's health care from the United Nations Population Fund (UNFPA). Then the United States became the only developed nation not to ratify the Convention on Elimination of All Forms of Discrimination Against Women.

Against all fact-based anecdotal and experiential information, the administration insisted that knowledge about sex encouraged promiscuity, mandating abstinence-only programs in schools. The administration limited vital information about birth control, even removing literature about condom effectiveness from the Department of Health and Human Services' website. Instead, they used the space to spread misinformation about abortion causing breast cancer and depression.

This was followed by a series of vastly restrictive acts: the charter of the Health and Human Services Secretary's Advisory Committee on Human Research Protection granted status as "human subjects" to embryos for the first time; the US House of Representatives passed legislation allowing health care entities to discriminate against any provider who even offered information about abortion; the president appointed anti-choice extremists to key FDA committees and to oversee Title X; and Congress prohibited the more than one hundred thousand women serving in the military and living on American bases overseas from obtaining abortion services in overseas military hospitals, even with their own money (to which Choices responded by offering abortions to military women at a reduced rate).

It was clear that the face of the war was changing once again. The combatants remained the same, but the nature of the attacks against women expanded into new territory. The Clinton era had seen a guerrilla war waged against abortion rights, with antis swarming abortion clinics, killing doctors, making overt threats, and ambushing patients on the streets. They had also begun chipping away at abortion rights incrementally with legislation and lawsuits in multiple states. These attacks were effective to a certain extent, but the antis lacked the main prize—the bully pulpit. When George W.

Bush took office, they won that, too. The antis no longer felt disenfranchised or alienated; now, the re-criminalization of abortion was much closer on the horizon. They leveraged their new support in the White House to help Bush fight what could only be described as a total war against reproductive freedom.

Women of the United States began falling prey to the quiet, carefully planned "stealth strategy" that characterized the Bush era. Realizing that the goal of overturning *Roe* remained elusive, the antis focused on achieving that same end by making it very difficult, and in some states almost impossible, to provide the procedure. The strategy had its roots in the 1992 US Supreme Court decision *Planned Parenthood v. Casey*, which declared for the first time that states had authority to regulate abortion clinics performing first trimester abortions (as opposed to only regulating those who provided second trimester abortions), as long as they didn't place an "undue burden" on women's access to abortions. The vague language of the ruling left states open to the antis' creative applications. They found ways to create small hurdles for clinics to climb if they wanted to stay in operation. Relatively benign on their own, these little obstacles piled up, making it more and more difficult for clinics to offer services. The goal was to create an environment where, in the words of one anti-choice leader, "abortion may indeed be perfectly legal, but no one can get one."

Their strategy was effective. Between 1995 and 2003, approximately 350 anti-choice measures were enacted, protecting pharmacists who refused to fill birth control prescriptions on moral or religious grounds, preventing physicians from performing most abortions, requiring state-controlled counseling and waiting periods for abortion, and mandating parental involvement in minors' abortions. There was also a rise in bogus malpractice cases brought against providers claiming that women were "coerced" into having abortions, and that many women didn't know they were actually "killing their babies." Most cases were dismissed or withdrawn, but each time a doctor was accused of malpractice, the ensuing legal fees and damage to the clinic's reputation did almost as much harm as if the cases had gone to trial.

Targeted Regulation of Abortion Provider (TRAP) Laws, designed to add excessive regulations and extra costs to abortion clinics, formed another arm of the total war campaign. States began requiring clinics to meet regulations that far exceeded the usual requirements of most medical facilities, including increased equipment, design, and training costs, higher licensing fees, and more documentation requirements. Some states mandated staffing levels above those usually needed for first-trimester abortions. New zoning ordinances were also passed to force clinics to move. They drove up the cost of abortions, placing them out of reach of many women, and forcing some clinics out of business.

During the Bush administration Choices had to change some of our practices, including rewording our consent forms, to conform to the new legal requirements. It was the most violative period of government interference in Choices' entire history. Aside from being licensed and regulated by New York State, Choices was also accredited by the Ambulatory Association of Health Care Centers (AAAHC), which gave us excellent reviews after inspecting the facility. But when the New York State Department of Health, which oversees the AAAHC regulators, came for an inspection one month later, their inspectors managed to find problems with the fire alarms, weak water pressure in two of our faucets, and gaps in our ceiling tiles—issues that were shared by the entire building, not just the clinic. Still, they threatened to close us down unless we made immediate repairs, which totaled approximately $400,000.

I had navigated such regulatory battles since Choices was still Flushing Women's, and I'd always found a way to survive. But many clinics simply could not manage the prohibitive cost of these attacks. The cost of abortions was always the one thing in health care that decreased. Patients received complete first trimester abortion care for under $400 dollars, a fee that had remained the same for twenty-five years. And since many providers often lowered their fees or waived them entirely for those in need, it became difficult, and sometimes impossible, to make ends meet. State by state, clinics began shutting down, until 87 percent of counties in the United States had no abortion providers.

One of the most maddening aspects of the stealth strategy was that it was conducted in the name of "women's health" in order to garner public support. Stricter regulations for clinics and laws mandating "unbiased" counseling were characterized as protections for women. The antis had found a new defense against accusations that they valued the fetus's life more than the mother's: turning the argument back on its head, they retorted that the mother and fetus had a sacred bond, and in honoring the "baby," they were also honoring the mother. They were slapping a women's rights label on fetal rights so that they could proclaim themselves women's rights activists, co-opting the language of feminism and thus pushing even more Americans to the anti-choice side of the reproductive rights continuum. Now, you could be "pro-life" and a feminist, too.

Pro-choice advocates were forced into a continually defensive posture. We lacked state power over the levers of government and we didn't have the support of powerful institutions like the Church, nor the millions of corporate dollars that were funneled into the right-to-life movement and the Republican party. The pro-choice movement literally lost ground every day as more clinics closed down and more Americans bought into the anti-choice vision. How could we fight against this multi-headed pro-life Hydra?

I thought perhaps the key lay in changing the legal foundation. *Roe* determined that the right to privacy under the Fourteenth Amendment's concept of personal liberty and restrictions upon state action was broad enough to encompass a woman's decision to terminate her pregnancy (within a gestational framework), thus classifying it as a fundamental right. But I had always believed that arguing for the right to reproductive freedom under the same umbrella as the right to read pornography in one's home was a tenuous arrangement. The US Constitution contains no express right to privacy, so the foundational legal pillar of women's reproductive freedom is vulnerable.

As I had written in my letter to Senator Hatch so many years ago, the right to reproductive freedom is as fundamental as the right not to be a slave. When birth control finally became available in all its forms, women's rights activists and feminists said that women were no longer slaves to their biology, that pregnancy would no longer be the guiding and primary directing principal of their lives. The legalization of abortion went even further toward freeing women from this constriction. In a sense it was a complete negation of the Freudian principle that "biology is destiny." But the ruling meant to uphold this right was full of holes inflicted state by state, its strength leaking out the sides. Now geography was destiny.

We needed a new starting place, a stronger legal base from which to articulate and ground our rights, one as airtight as laws against slavery. As the stealth laws threatened to defeat the impact of *Roe*, I became more and more convinced that the right to abortion should have been articulated under the Thirteenth Amendment. This would frame reproductive freedom as a universal human right, and perhaps give the pro-choice movement the strength to hold the relentless attacks by the antis at bay.

The matter became even more urgent when President Bush dropped another bomb in 2003, signing into law the Partial Birth Abortion Ban Act, the first legislation to criminalize an abortion procedure since *Roe v. Wade*. The law forbade the procedure even if a woman's health was endangered, mandated prison terms and financial penalties for doctors who recommended abortions, and allowed a woman's male partner or parents to sue her if she had the procedure against their will. Planned Parenthood and two other organizations sued the government, and the ban was struck down by three federal district courts, but this unprecedented attack was the most audacious yet against *Roe*.

Outraged by this blatant disrespect for women's rights and well-being, I brought my ideas to a Veteran Feminists of America event honoring Justice Ruth Bader Ginsburg. I wanted to hear her opinion on whether or not lawyers should be working toward recasting reproductive freedom as part of the Thirteenth Amendment. "I have criticized the Court's decision in *Roe v. Wade*—not, of course, for the result," Ginsberg replied when I asked her my question. "I think the notion [is] that it isn't just some private act; it is a woman's right to control her own life." *Roe* had made abortion legal, but it was not strong enough to cast reproductive freedom as a positive moral value.

The morality of the decision had been defined by the religious class. Even people who supported the right to abortion said that despite abortion being legal, and possibly the best decision under the circumstances, it would never really be objectively moral; it would never be a purely positive good. Women making the decision remained suspects or victims at best, and murderers at worst. Saying "I had an abortion" aloud hadn't gotten any easier since 1973. Abortion was ever a tragedy, a necessary evil, something to be kept private and about which to feel ashamed.

As long as people see abortion as immoral, its legality will be in danger. How, then, to move beyond the legality and embrace the morality? How to fully combine the two and produce ethical laws? How to create a transcendent class of women as active moral agents with which people identify and will fight to defend? The future of abortion still comes down to that fundamental question: Can we really have abortion without apology?

Women must gain the kind of biological entitlement (and the sense of power and agency) that comes so much more easily to men. To secure reproductive freedom as a fundamental right and abortion as a moral choice, we must forge our own paths to selfhood. And with these selves, we must create and assent to laws and cultural norms that serve us and withdraw consent to those that do not. As Sojourner Truth said, "If women want any rights more than they's got, why don't they just take them, and not be talking about it?" Why, indeed.

The movement was too quiet. There was little coordinated pro-choice activism. The main theater of battle was the courts, where consistent legal defense was necessary to attempt to block the cascade of restrictions that were proposed. NARAL, NOW, the Feminist Majority, and Planned Parenthood—the main pro-choice institutions—remained in the front of the firing lines, but they continued to lose both legal battles and the hearts and minds of many women.

Meanwhile, the clinics struggled on, and the patients kept coming.

THE GOING WAS TOUGH at Choices. I had been glad to help support people who needed help after 9/11 through the Mental Health Center, but the massive legal fees I had incurred in recent years made the continued subsidy of Mental Health Center expenses impossible. In order for me to keep Choices running, I had to disband the center after ten years of operation. I had created something that was very dear to me, but I had also learned when to let go.

Riding horses, that beloved pastime that had given me solace through the worst trials of my life, also faded into the past. I endured several traumatic injuries to my hips, and the pain became so excruciating that I began to have difficulty walking and bending. I was finally forced to have hip replacement surgery. By then I'd sold Garrison and donated all twenty-seven of my animals to good homes. I moved to East Hampton and brought only Hollywould. I kept her at a stable in East Hampton for a couple of years, but it was becoming more and more obvious that I would never really be able to ride again.

After fully recovering from my surgery, I went with Mahin for a summer weekend retreat to the Otesaga Hotel in Cooperstown. I'd spent so many summers of my childhood in the country, at overnight camps where the days were hot and steamy and the nights required cool clothing. But this was the first summer that I had embraced since my childhood, the first summer I felt so powerfully the passing of time, the first time I anticipated greeting the first coloring of the leaves in the fall with alarm. The first time I felt I was aging. I was beginning to feel that so much of my life was behind me.

I took a trip to Normandy to walk the massive beaches with their history of blood and battles. I stopped in Caen, where the young Charlotte Corday had grown up, and then went on to Rouen, where Joan of Arc was tried and burned. I entered a small museum and walked down a winding set of stairs to a room filled with *tableaux vivants* of famous stages of Joan's career. I rested in front of each one, relishing my past imaginings, when a young family with a son about five years old came in behind me. The parents stood with their child between them, pointing to scenes in the montage, teaching, showing—a transmission of cultural memory before my eyes.

How would it feel, I thought, to have a little girl next to me right now?

That night, I wrote in my journal:

I pick up this novel—Kaddish for an Unborn Child, by Imre Kertész—and by the third page I am crying, because I know I will be faced with thinking about it—no, not thinking about it—feeling it. Feeling that question, that question without answer, the question that I always answered so glibly, so matter of factly: What would my child have been like if I hadn't had an abortion?

There is an answer inside me. It came out the night before the abortion, the night I wrote "For one night I am a mother."

Of course I'd thought about this unborn child before, but I would only allow myself fleeting encounters with the fantasy of being a mother. I imagined a small, intense girl walking beside me on the beach, the whitecaps moving in horizontal lines while our footprints made matching patterns in the sand. But I would quickly put these thoughts away, forgetting her for months at a time. After all, I was busy with the reality I had chosen, and it had never included a child.

Now, at age fifty-eight, I allowed myself to think about what had always seemed impossible. I wanted a child. I wanted a daughter.

At first, this intense desire would come in waves and beat at the shores of my heart and then subside, leaving me with only a memory of the storm. I tried to be realistic, going over exactly how I would have to change my life in order to incorporate a child. For so long I couldn't imagine making these changes. Then the desire took hold of me with such a compelling force that I felt like I had succumbed to a tsunami. It was a moment of grace, an epiphany, a gift. It was the culmination of so much of my life, a setting free. I was going to adopt a little girl.

I reasoned I probably had at least twenty years left. If I lived to seventy-eight, then she would be twenty-five years old, the age that I was when my father died. Would the years that I had left be enough to give her a good foundation? Would I be able to integrate her into a life built totally around my own rhythms? How would it feel to be a mother? Would I like her? Would I love her? How would it feel for her? Would she like me, love me?

I had known many of love's faces. I had been consumed by passion, loved tenderly, possessively, and selfishly. But I had never loved unconditionally, the way parental love is described. And it came to me that the little girl I would adopt had not experienced limitless love either. Perhaps she had not experienced love at all—only its pale shadow through her caretakers. Strangers to this reality, we would have to find our way together. I found this thought strangely comforting, as if I would be adopting a comrade-in-arms.

My only experience with human adoption had been at Choices. Occasionally I'd receive adoption requests with photos of happy and seemingly well-adjusted white families desperate to have a child, and willing to pay for one. I could not imagine asking a woman to keep a pregnancy she did not want for $10,000 or a million dollars. It would be akin to asking her to set a price on her freedom or on her free will. I wanted to adopt someone already born, waiting, alone, unwanted and abandoned.

I initially thought of adopting a Chinese girl, since the Chinese were notorious for one-child-only policies, sex selection abortions, and ubiquitous female infanticide. But in truth, I was not confident that I could deal with raising a child of a different race, with all the added complications that brings. I thought I could minimize the challenges by having a child with my heritage in common. Since Russia was so much a part of me, it seemed natural to go there.

I knew that taking a child out of a foreign orphanage was a huge risk. AIDS, fetal alcohol syndrome—I'd heard the tragic stories of adoptions gone horribly wrong. I wanted a child I could raise, but not an infant. There could be too many potential medical problems that wouldn't have manifested themselves in the early stages of development, and I knew I could not take on the responsibility of a special needs child. After much research and many discussions with Mahin, I decided that a three-year-old would be the best fit.

I began the adoption proceedings.

ONE YEAR LATER my plane to Russia lurched in the icy darkness. Anxiety engulfed me as I looked at the white whirlwind outside my window. Now, by adopting, was I admitting that something was missing? Had I fallen into that essentialist hole of thinking that no matter what a woman does, she will not be a complete woman until she has a child? Was this the actualization of all my becoming—or a final existential crisis of meaning?

Hurtling through the sky to meet my little girl, I forced my thoughts to stop racing. I knew the answers. The decision to adopt her had come as organically as the decision to create Patient Power, to build Choices, to expand to Russia, to breathe freely and live my life as a fully realized individual. These acts were all results of a process of decision making of which I was hardly conscious. The fact that I was fifty-eight? Well, it had taken me that long to be ready. I was ready.

The day after my arrival in Moscow, I drove to Children's Home Number 13, where my little girl was a numbered and filed ward of the Russian state. She was three years and two months old. She had blonde hair and blue eyes. Her birth date was September 26, 2001. Her name was Irena, which, I was told, meant "peace" in Russian. That was all I knew about her when I pulled up in front of the orphanage.

For the adoption to proceed on schedule, I had to make a decision by the end of the week. After that, I'd return to New York for two or three months until Irena was available for official adoption. I, who had made so many decisions in so many crisis situations, found myself humbled. As with abortion, this was a lifelong, irrevocable decision. Whatever the intended or unintended consequences were, I had to live with them permanently. This child would live with them, too. I was making a decision that would not only change my life forever, but hers. The power and audacity of it all took my breath away.

I opened the door and heat rushed at me. The smells were wet and institutional, like a New York City public hospital. Inside, I was met with pure Russian bureaucracy: filling out papers, waiting, and filling out more papers. After what seemed an endless amount of time, the director finally approached me. "Would you like to have tea or immediately proceed to meet Irena?"

I turned and saw a part of her for the first time. She was peeking out from behind an adult arm, wearing two of those classic crunched bows people put on top of the heads of little girls. She was crying and rubbing her eyes with her fists.

"Irenitchka, go say hello to Mama," the director told her. She came over to me and put her little thin arms around my neck. There was hardly any weight to her touch. I held her tight against me as she whimpered, "Ma Ma Ma Ma."

Had they told her that her mother finally had come to get her? What would they tell her if I didn't want to adopt her after all? Did she have any idea of how high the stakes were? In her own child's way was she attempting to be the best little girl she could so she would be chosen? My heart froze at the thought of her potential level of performance anxiety.

She already had a life, a reference group to which she was attached. Was this her family? Would she miss them? There were approximately twenty children in her group with only one other girl. I learned that it was not unusual for parents to put their children in orphanages because they could not afford to feed them—another casualty of the breakup of the Soviet Union. These were the children who were not aborted between the twelfth and the fifteenth or the thirty-fifth abortion. They called every caretaker Mama. Most would likely never be adopted. Would it have been better for them to be aborted? I knew their future: bleak prostitution for many of the girls, drunken unemployment for the boys.

When I walked with Irena into the playroom the other children crowded near me, tried to sit on my lap, called me Mama, looked up at me with wanting eyes. Irena blocked them, already proprietary. I stroked her thin hair in those two big bows. I saw that she was practically bald in the back of her head. They told me it was because she moved her head back and forth on her pillow at night, a typical orphanage self-soothing behavior pattern to help her sleep.

She went to the couch, stood on it, and lifted up the curtain, pointing outside and saying, "Sobaka. Sobaka." Dog. I saw a small mutt who seemed to live there. I laughed and took out a photo of my dog Pushkin, saying, "This is my Sobaka." Irena looked at the picture and then turned again to the window to show me hers. "Sobaka doggie," I said. She repeated it. I had created a common word—a common world.

I SPENT THE WEEK visiting Irena every day until the time came to decide. Her caretakers told me how much more engaged and responsive she had become since meeting me.

I could see it in her eyes. Now that she had found me, she was probably wondering if I would keep her. I tried to imagine her three-year-old consciousness. What must it be like to be so helpless, so powerless? Even though all children experience powerlessness in different degrees, hers was so absolute.

This child, abandoned at birth—unwanted. Her skin was too dry, speech too delayed, her mother too young and too poor. Was Irena the result of the mother's first real love, a one-night stand, a rape or a trick? What act of desperation led her mother to abandon the premature baby girl in the hospital where she would spend the first two months of her life in the intensive care unit?

"Do you want to proceed with this referral?" the director asked.

Others were in the room, but I felt alone. "Yes, I want to proceed. Yes. I do." I felt dizzy with the decision. I changed my life and embraced my fate.

The director asked me what name she was to be called. At this moment I felt a sense of possession: this is my child, and

I must give her a name. I had come to Russia with the idea of naming my daughter Sasha. I spontaneously combined Sasha and Irena and said, "Sasharina." It sounded magical and musical and flexible. The caretakers found the name beautiful. I had created something new that would become part of our legend.

On the last day of my trip, as I said goodbye for now, I gave Sasharina my picture. "Ya vernoos," I told her. I will return. She surprised all of us when she held the picture out with both hands and placed it against her heart. Then she kissed it. I was profoundly moved by this expression. No tribute in the past or in the future could ever equal this one. I thought, "This is how love begins."

BACK HOME, thoughts of becoming a mother crowded out the obsessive worry about liquidating pensions and investments to keep Choices going during what was becoming a very difficult financial bind. However anxious I was, I believed in my ability to turn it all around. I had a daughter now. I had someone who gave me more than myself to survive for.

I called family and friends and caught them up on the details of the trip. Some listened in wide-eyed amazement, while others expressed anxiety about their losing priority in my orbit and my being too old. To my dismay my twenty-year friendship with Phyllis ended. It became obvious that she did not have the desire or will to deal with my having a child. It was deeply disappointing, but I couldn't dwell on it. Like marriage, divorce, and death, having children restructures one's relationships.

Other friends were supportive. The sculptor Linda Stein invited me to a political gathering for History in Action, a listserv for Second and Third Wave feminists. I walked into her loft in Soho and recognized a young journalist, Jennifer

Baumgardner, who had done direct action work on the abortion issue. She was visibly pregnant, and I made my way over to her to share my "pregnancy." Later that evening I surprised myself (and everyone there who knew me) even more. When Linda got up in front of the room to welcome everyone, she asked me to come up and say something. In the past, I would have thanked her and presented some political issue or action for everyone to think about. This time, I began with the words, "I have just returned from Siberia . . . I am a mother."

Yet I had to laugh at my current version of motherhood. Before I left Omsk, I had made arrangements to speak with Sasha a couple of times a week over the phone. It was the only way I could think of to keep some kind of connection with her. Now, I found myself standing in my kitchen at 3 a.m. saying, "Sasha, sobaka-doggie" and "Ya vernoos." Sasha didn't respond to this. The only thing I heard back was the sound of screaming children and then silence as the calls dropped.

I called my attorney and changed my will to include my daughter. And of course I went shopping for everything that I thought she and I might need. The consumer landscape of motherhood was all encompassing—clothing, toys, DVDs, sheets, furniture—an endless sea of colorful inanimate objects.

The director of the orphanage had mentioned that the building needed new flooring in the main room and new curtains in another. I arranged to take care of this, thinking of Sasha's friends who would be left behind. The time passed with preparations and my labors of love. In these small and big ways, my life changed.

WHEN I RETURNED to Russia to get Sasharina, I entered the orphanage purposefully. I stuck my head into the door of the playroom and stretched my neck to look for her. I saw a little blonde head turning to look for me, then her face, filled with recognition. Her eyes shouted, "You have returned!" Sasha rushed to meet me as I opened my arms wide. I felt every part of her smiling as I swept her up into my arms and held her tight against me.

The audience of caretakers watched as the other children gathered around us. My arms were not wide enough to hold all the need, and my heart broke a little with the attempt to stretch it. The orphanage receded as our car pulled away and we watched as the kids outside ran toward the car, waving to us, their figures fading in the snow. Sasha sat quietly. I thought how utterly small and vulnerable she was. I put my arm around her and she leaned against me.

I brought Sasha up to our hotel room, alone together for the first time. She immediately morphed into a whirling dervish, running through the rooms, jumping on and off the bed, turning light switches on and off. I tried to lay her down on the bed and the pillows started flying. She was scared. I was overwhelmed, frustrated, tired, and getting angry. I managed to place a call to Mahin. "What do I do?"

She said, "Just *hold* her."

I realized that Sasha was having an acute anxiety attack. Whatever could her three-year-old mind make of all this? She had been taken away from all the security and familiarity she had ever known, barraged with new sights, sounds, and terrifying large spaces with this woman who spoke strange words and tried to hold her. It must have been some kind of nightmare.

I went into the bedroom with her, closed the door, and turned off the lights. We lay down on the bed and I held her next to me. She screamed and thrashed. She tried to push me away. "Shh . . . it's alright," I told her. "Sasha, shh—try and sleep. I won't hurt you."

She finally fell asleep, exhausted.

The last night we were in Moscow, I took Sasha to Red Square. It was snowing lightly. The cupolas of St. Basil's Cathedral rose to the black sky in fantastic shapes and colors like snow cones. We basked in the moment, and I knew that one day I would be back here with her.

She was wild again in the airport. We were late for our flight. I found a cart, lifted Sasha, put her in the pullout where pocketbooks are usually kept, placed the luggage on the bottom, and began to run. Racing through the airport to get to the gate, she put her arms out like a bird and made flying motions, screaming with delight. I passed escalators, reading signage at warp speed as I yelled, "Excuse me! Excuse me!" My chest felt like it was going to explode. I had to make this flight to New York.

Finally, we arrived at the security section for our gate. I tried to catch my breath, but Sasha ran in and out through the metal detectors. I followed her, setting off the alarms with my metal hip. I stopped to reorganize our bags, and when I looked up, Sasha was gone. I looked around and saw an older woman leaning over her. She brought Sasha over to me and asked, "Is this your daughter?"

"Yes," I said as I tried to hold onto Sasha.

"She says she doesn't have a mother."

I felt as if I had been punched in the stomach and struggled to gain control. It was too much to explain, so I simply thanked the woman for catching her.

FEBRUARY 15, 2006. It was our family's anniversary—two years from the day Sasha came to New York with me. I took her out to dinner and sang "Happy Anniversary" to the tune of "Happy Birthday," which was her favorite song (birthdays were not celebrated in the orphanage). Mahin sat next to her and told her the story of her homecoming. There would come a day when she would ask for a more complete story, for me to tell her where she came from and why she was here. I would tell her as much as I knew.

As I put Sasha to bed later that night, she smiled. "I know who you are," she said.

"Who am I?"

"You are my mother."

"Yes. And you are my daughter."

She laughed. After two years, she was beginning to trust this, and so was I. We had found each other. I was Sasha's home, and she was mine.

My mother and Murray, her companion for thirty-five years now, formed part of our home, too, when they came to visit me shortly after I adopted Sasha. My mother had been going blind for the last three years with macular degeneration, and I could gauge the level of her declining sight by the nuances of her critique of me. "Your ass is too wide," she used to say. "Your breasts are showing. Why are you wearing flat shoes? You should dye your hair blonde again." Now she just touched me and told me how much she loved me, her frail hands embracing me while her clouded eyes searched my face. Oddly, I missed the criticism. This new expression of love felt somehow inauthentic.

But watching my mother get to know and love Sasha, I felt my love for her change. For the first time I experienced the joy of family and a true sense of being home. I thought of the moment I'd brought Sasha home to meet my mother. I'd slowed the car, wanting to freeze the moment of anticipation, to hold it forever. Sasha ran across the lawn as my mother watched from the window . . . and then she was in my mother's arms, my mother, my daughter, then me. My mother had always had problems giving and receiving, but here was a gift that was defined by the giving. With Sasha there were no boundaries, and now the boundaries to my love for my mother also dissolved. I watched the light in my mother's eyes as she held Sasha tightly and kissed her with passionate force, laughing loudly at Sasha's funny antics and mothering her in a way I did not remember experiencing myself.

She became ill with Alzheimer's. She was afraid she would be put away, and no amount of reassurance would convince her otherwise. When she began to die, I went to stay with her in Florida. In the pain and struggle of her oncoming death, I found more warmth and intensity than ever before. I was her daughter, her sister, her mother, and her friend. As I held her in my arms, her childishness became a bittersweet burden. I diapered her, fed her, gave her medication, soothed her when she cried out, kissed her all over. I sensed memories of the time I existed within her body. I was holding her in her hospital bed at home when she began to turn into a corpse, her beloved Chopin waltzes and nocturnes playing on the CD player. It was the most intimate and loving interaction I ever had with her.

A FEW DAYS LATER, I sat in my house on the bay, eagerly awaiting the sunrise. I wrote as I looked for the light of dawn. I was no longer afraid of death. I said yes to life because that is all we know. And living with Sasha made the whole experience bigger, almost epic, and at the same time intimate, sacred, and precious.

Sasha would carry me into the future. I was a mother, and all the philosophical questions of my life were now played out in the smallest of places. I knew there would be no lack of battles for her to fight in the generational struggle for women's rights. As my ancestors had done for me, I would instill in her a sense of romance in revolution. I would teach her that it is never purely a cerebral or theoretical process, although analysis can give it form and direction. Revolution at its core is driven by love.

I took Sasha with me to Choices sometimes. Outside the entrance, we'd see dependable Sister Dorothy, still standing outside the front doors handing out rosaries and pink plastic fetuses in rain or shine after all these years. We would nod "good mornings" when we saw each other, but we never really entered into conversation until she found out that I had adopted a child. She began to give me children's books, little Bible stories that I accepted but did not use. Aware of my love of philosophy, she even gave me a copy of "Purity of Heart is to Will One Thing," the famous treatise in which Kierkegaard writes of the responsibility of single-minded spiritual seeking, offering clues to the nature of the good while insisting that each of us find it for ourselves. Though I never forgot that she was the enemy of everything I held sacred, I was touched by her gesture.

One day when I stopped to chat with her outside the clinic, I shared with Sister Dorothy how much I loved being a mother. She smiled. "I am sure you are a good mother. But you would be a better one if you stopped killing all those little Sashas in there."

At that moment I was filled with absolute certainty of the one true thing I knew: that there were women and girls who were waiting for my help that day and for the foreseeable future, and that this war to stop me and others from doing that would never end in my lifetime. I was grateful to play my part and I had learned to love the struggle.

Sasha took my hand. Together we turned and walked into Choices.

Acknowledgments

MY FIRST THANKS go to three women deeply loved and so recently lost: Ruth Hoffman (1917–2008), Mahin Hassibi (1937–2009), and Cynthia Colquitt-Craven (1941–2009). Vividly present by their absence, they infused my creative process with demands for clarity and truth.

My deepest appreciation to family and friends whose love, support, and just being there have been invaluable to me: Michael Dubow, for being a loving anchor and wise counsel; Diane Dubow, for gently accepting our differences; Jackie Rovine, for her ambition and psychological courage; Lisa Norton, for her empathy and reinforcement; Carolee Lucenti, for always laughing and forgiving; Linda Stein, for her vision and love; Vaughna Feary, for her wisdom and guidance; Andrea Peyser, for her wit and solidarity; Bill Baird, for sharing the front lines and lifelong support; and Stanley Rustin, for being the psychological bookends of my life—my trusted, loving witness.

I want to express my gratitude to my staff at Choices, the

doctors, nurses, and administration who have made it possible not only to do the work we do but also to survive and write about it. Thanks especially to Dr. Lorna Aguilos, for her loyalty, persistence, and belief in the mission; to Carmine Asparro, for being an ally, friend, and guru through the most difficult of times; and to Annette Farrell, for sharing the growth, struggles, and triumphs of Choices for so many years and coming back for more.

This book is also an offering to my patients. The work, the mission, and this book would never have been possible without the thousands and thousands of women and girls who have come to Choices through all the years in trust and hope. Their persistence and dignity in the face of obstacles, violence, and harassment are a testament to their courage. Quiet heroines all, it is a privilege and a gift to have spent my life serving them.

Much appreciation goes to all the writers, activists, and editors at *On the Issues Magazine*, who have assisted me in creating the voice of a visionary, progressive feminism—particularly my extraordinary editor Cindy Cooper who shares my passion for reproductive justice; Mark Phillips, for his creative and technological brilliance; Mary Lou Greenberg, for always being there with me on the front and written lines in the struggle for abortion rights; and to Vanessa Valenti, my social marketing guru.

Particular thanks to Jennifer Baumgardner, for being able to share the struggles of the movement, the joy of our children, and for creating the initial outline for this book. My first editor, reader, and longtime ally, she was instrumental in bringing this book to life.

Special thanks to my archivist Laura Micham at the Sallie Bingham Center for Women's History and Culture at Duke University, for her consistent public support of my work.

Her assistance with the research for this project has been invaluable.

My deep appreciation to Florence Howe for her pioneering vision in creating the Feminist Press. My book could not have found a better home. Many thanks to executive director Gloria Jacobs for strongly believing in this project and having the courage to use the A word. Much gratitude and admiration to my dear friend Blanche Wiesen Cook for her long friendship and early consistent support for this project.

This book would not be possible without the creative political intelligence, razor-sharp instincts, and feel for my particular literary rhythm of Feminist Press editorial director Amy Scholder—it has been a rare privilege working with her. Thanks also to the staff of the Feminist Press, Drew Stevens, Sophie Hagen, Jeanann Pannasch, and Elizabeth Koke for their assistance in this process.

And special, deep, and enduring appreciation to Theresa Noll, my editor who worked intimately with me for two years helping craft a form and narrative arc onto the whirlwind of my life. She was a gentle navigator, drawing me into my past and away from my own resistance.

And of course eternal gratitude to my daughter Sasharina —North Star of my autumn, who is forever challenging and delighting me.

And finally to Elizabeth Tudor (a.k.a. Queen Elizabeth I of England), for serving as my imaginary companion and role model for as long as I can remember.

Notes

1. Lizza, "The Abortion Capital of America."
2. Carole Joffe's *Doctors of Conscience: The Struggle to Provide Abortion Before and After Roe v. Wade* is an excellent account of doctors who risked everything to help women in need.
3. See Hoffman, "Isn't It Enough To Make You Scream?"
4. Patient Power, which planted the seeds of the medical consumer movement, was far in advance of its time. It has taken years for the notion that patients have rights to take root in public consciousness, much less law, but recently that has begun to change. Second opinions have become generalized, alternative treatments are available, there are multiple patient advocacy groups, and doctors are rated on the Internet according to patient criteria. The New York State Department of Health has a set of guidelines called the "Patient Bill of Rights" requiring medical facilities to establish policies regarding the rights of patients and ensuring that all patients are informed of

their rights and responsibilities. Health Insurance Portability and Accountability Act (HIPPA) requirements protect patient privacy. The Advisory Commission on Consumer Protection and Quality in the Health Care Industry was formed in 1997 to "advise the president on changes occurring in the health care system and recommend measures as may be necessary to promote and assure health care quality and value, and protect consumers and workers in the health care system." As part of its work, Clinton asked the Commission to draft a "consumer bill of rights" (see "Consumer Bill of Rights and Responsibilities"). And in June of 2010 the Obama administration released the "Fact Sheet: The Affordable Care Act's New Patient's Bill of Rights" to help Americans navigate their health care coverage ("The Obama Administration's New 'Patient's Bill Of Rights'"). In the case of doctors being gods, one could definitely make the argument that this particular god is dead.

5. Not long after, Rosie Jimenez, a twenty-seven-year-old single mother too poor to pay for the procedure at a private clinic, had an illegal and unsafe abortion. She became the first of many women to die as a result of the Hyde Amendment. At a 1979 meeting held by abortion rights leaders Gloria Steinem, Karen Mulhauser of NARAL, and Uta Landy of NAF, Ellen Frankfort, coauthor of *Rosie: Investigation of a Wrongful Death,* announced the formation of the Rosie Jimenez Fund, the first to provide direct subsidy for women seeking abortions without sufficient funds to pay for one.

6. As of today, there are only four states that voluntarily provide Medicaid funding for abortions.

7. This eventually became a double-edged sword as the state began to use the system of regulation and licensing

to control and eliminate providers through TRAP laws (see chapter nine).

8. I went on to hold a second panel on women's health in 1976. This one was sponsored by the Medical Group Council (Marty was the chairman) and titled "'Challenging the Medical Mystique': How Can Consumers Influence the Health Care Delivery System?" May Lasker, Philip Strax, and Congressman Leo Zeferetti were participants.

9. Menstrual extraction is a method of self-help abortion that was developed and implemented by Lorraine Rothman and Carol Downer at the Feminist Women's Health Center in 1971. It is a manually-operated suction technique using tubes and syringe that can be performed by lay people without medical expertise. Rothman and Downer called the technique ME to emphasize its innocuous use in suctioning out menstrual blood and tissue. ME was also considered an important tactical weapon in the abortion wars; if *Roe* were ever overturned, or states started to substantially restrict access, women would still be able to control their fertility.

10. Ross, "Abortion: Six Years After the Supreme Court Decision, The Conflict Rages On."

11. *Bellotti v. Baird* was argued twice and ruled on after its 1979 hearing. The case involved a Massachusetts law that required minor girls seeking abortions to first obtain the consent of their parents, or a court order waiving that consent. The court's eight-to-one decision in 1979 affirmed its previous ruling in *Danforth*, invalidating all state laws that require all minor girls to obtain their parents' consent before getting an abortion. It gave states latitude to establish procedures to determine whether a girl is mature enough to make the decision. But it held

that a pregnant minor is "entitled in such a proceeding to show either that she is mature enough and well enough informed to make her abortion decision, in consultation with her physician, independently of her parents' wishes," or that the abortion would be in her "best interest."

12. FDA studies from the early eighties showed that of one hundred women who use aerosol foam alone, two to twenty-nine became pregnant in the first year; of those who used jellies and cream alone, four to thirty-six became pregnant. . . . When compared to the pill (two to three out of one hundred users became pregnant in a year), IUD (one to six) and the diaphragm (two to twenty, depending on proper use), the nonprescription spermicides seemed much less effective. (See Hoffman, "Birth Control: The Last Market That Needs Misleading Ads.")

13. See Frances Kissling, "If War is 'Just', So is Abortion." Also see Judith Jarvis Thomson's famous philosophical tract *A Defense of Abortion* (1971).

14. Erlanger, "A Widening Pattern of Abuse Exemplified in Steinberg Case."

15. Faludi, *Backlash*.

16. Members included CARASA, Catholics for a Free Choice, Choices, NYS-NARAL, NOW-NYC, Planned Parenthood-NYC, Radical Women, Religious Coalition for Abortion Rights, the Women's Quarterly Review, Hunter College, the Puerto Rican Committee Against Racism, the Local 3882 AFT Organization of Asian Women, and Princeton University. Among many others, the individual members included Charlotte Bunch, Rhonda Copelon, Kate Millett, Grace Paley, Phyllis Chesler, Bella Abzug, and Ruth Messinger.

17. Benderly, "Feminists Fight Fundamentalist "Fetus Fetish."

18. Ibid.

19. See Shelley, "A Sacrificial Light, Self-Immolation in Tajr-ish Square, Tehran," for more on this subject.

20. Robin Morgan later hit this nail on the head with her book *Sisterhood Is Global: The International Women's Movement Anthology*.

21. Recipients of Diana Foundation grants included Andrea Dworkin, for her book *Scapegoat*; NOW of New York City; The House of Elder Artists (THEA); Community Health Care Network; Phyllis Chesler; and Edna Adan Ismail, director and founder of the Edna Adan University Hospital in Hargeisa and president of the Organization for Victims of Torture.

22. Karl Marx, from "Critique of the Gotha Program."

23. Patrick Buchanan, one of the Republican candidates for President, told four hundred people at a New Jersey right-to-life convention that "the empire we are fighting is every bit the evil empire the Soviet Union was" (see Hoffman, "Abortion Providers: The New 'Communists,'" in *On the Issues*).

24. I first met Norma McCorvey at the second national Pro-Choice March on Washington in 1989. She greeted me with a wan smile as activist lawyer Gloria Allred intro-duced her first as Norma McCorvey and then as "you know, Jane Roe."

25. The *New York Times*, January 11, 1999: "GOLD-Martin, M.D., 80 years old, died the kind of death, in Fort Lau-derdale, Florida, on January 9, 1999, that he had always termed a 'blessing'—one that came quickly and without great suffering. The lessons of his life can be measured by his achievements in the medical world and the gifts of loving compassion and generosity that he shared with all who knew him. As a physician, he practiced the art

as well as the science of medicine, and his patients loved him for it. As a mentor, he inspired many young professionals to move beyond their limitations and live their dreams. As a man, he was honorable, honest, loving, witty, and kind. He will be deeply missed and very fondly remembered by his loving wife, Merle Hoffman . . ."

Works Cited

A complete archive of Merle Hoffman's *On the Issues* magazine editorials and interviews, as well as her writing on current feminist topics, can be found at ontheissuesmagazine .com. See merlehoffman.com for further resources on Merle's life and activism.

Advancing New Standards In Reproductive Health. 2010. *Fetal pain, analgesia, and anesthesia in the context of abortion.* ANSIRH, June. http://www.ansirh.org/_documents/ research/late-abortion/FetalPain.FactSheet.6-2010.pdf

Baird-Windle, Patricia and Eleanor Bader. 2001. *Targets of Hatred: Anti-Abortion Terrorism.* New York: Palgrave Macmillan.

Benderly, Jill. 1986. "Feminists Fight Fundamentalist 'Fetus Fetish.'" *New York Guardian*, February 5.

Branch, Alan. 2004. "Radical Feminism and Abortion Rights: A Brief Summary and Critique." *JBMW* 9, no. 2 (Fall).

Epstein, Richard A. 1993. "Life's Dominion: An Argument About Abortion, Euthanasia, and Individual Freedom." *Reason,* November 1. http://www.highbeam.com/doc/1G1-14527043.html

Erlanger, Steven. 1987. "A Widening Pattern of Abuse Exemplified in Steinberg Case." *New York Times,* November 8.

Faludi, Susan. 1992. *Backlash: The Undeclared War Against American Women.* New York: Anchor.

Fine, Terri Susan. 2006. "Generations, Feminist Beliefs and Abortion Rights Support." *Journal of International Women's Studies* 7, no. 4 (May). http://facta.junis.ni.ac.rs/lal/lal2009/lal2009-12.pdf

Gowaty, Patricia Adair, ed. 1997. *Feminism and Evolutionary Biology: Boundaries, Intersections, and Frontiers.* New York: Chapman & Hall.

Grimes, David A. 1991. "An Epidemic of Antiabortion Violence in the United States." *American Journal of Obstetrics and Gynecology* 165, no. 5 (November).

Guttmacher Institute. 2006. "Abortion and Unintended Pregnancy Decline Worldwide as Contraceptive Use Increases." Media release. http://www.guttmacher.org/media/nr/2009/10/13/index.html

Hern, Warren M., MD. 1972. "The Politics Of Abortion." *The Progressive* 36, no. 11 (November).

Hewson, Barbara. 2004. "Is It Murder To Refuse A Caesarean?" *AIMS Journal* 16, no. 1 (Spring). http://www.aims.org.uk/Journal/Vol16No1/murderToRefuse.htm

Hoffman, Amy. 2001. "A Conversation With Abortion Rights Activist Merle Hoffman." *Wellesley Review.*

Hoffman, Merle. 1982. "Birth Control: The Last Market That Needs Misleading Ads." *Los Angeles Times,* August 29.

———. 1985. "Feminism, Power, Politics, Abortion." *Journal of The American Medical Women's Association* 40, no. 6 (November/December).

Joffe, Carole E. 1995. *Doctors of Conscience: The Struggle to Provide Abortion Before and After* Roe v. Wade. Boston: Beacon Press.

Kissling, Frances. 1991. "If War Is 'Just', So Is Abortion." *Los Angeles Times*, April 17.

Lee, Clara N., and John M. Daly. 2002. "Provider Volume and Clinical Outcomes in Surgery: Issues and Implications." *Bulletin of the American College of Surgeons* 86, no. 6 (June).

Lewin, Tamar. 1995. "A New Weapon in an Old War—A Special Report; Latest Tactic Against Abortion: Accusing Doctors of Malpractice." *New York Times*, April 9.

Lizza, Ryan. 2005. "The Abortion Capital of America." *New York Times Magazine*, December 4.

McKenna, George. 1995. "On Abortion: A Lincolnian Position." *Atlantic Monthly*, September.

Meikle, James. 2010. "Human Foetus Feels No Pain Before 24 Weeks, Study Says." *Guardian*, June 25. http://www.guardian.co.uk/lifeandstyle/2010/jun/25/human-foetus-no-pain-24-weeks

Morgan, Robin. 1996. *Sisterhood Is Global: The International Women's Movement Anthology*. New York: The Feminist Press.

Murray, Alice. 1981. "A Survey On Abortion Finds Its Illegality Would Not Deter 45% Of Women." *Daily News*, November 22.

Pollitt, Katha. 1997. "Abortion in American History." *Atlantic Monthly*, May. http://www.theatlantic.com/issues/97may/abortion.htm

Pollitt, Katha. 1997. "Secrets And Lies." *Nation*, March 31.

Rich, Frank. 1997. "Partial-Truth Abortion." *New York Times*, March 9.

Ross, Barbara. 1979. "Abortion: Six Years After the Supreme Court Decision, the Conflict Rages On." *New York Post,* February 13.

Sarachild, Kathie, Carol Hanisch, Faye Levine, Barbara Leon, and Colette Price, eds. 1979. *Feminist Revolution: An Abridged Edition With Additional Writings.* New York: Random House.

Shelley, Martha. 1994. "A Sacrificial Light: Self-Immolation in Tajrish Square, Tehran." *On the Issues,* Fall.

Smith-Rosenberg, Carroll. 1985. *Disorderly Conduct: Visions of Gender in Victorian America.* New York: Alfred A. Knopf.

Solinger, Rickie. 2001. *Beggars and Choosers: How the Politics of Choice Shapes Adoption, Abortion, and Welfare in the United States.* New York: Farrar, Straus and Giroux.

Staggenborg, Suzanne. 1994. *The Pro-Choice Movement: Organization and Activism in the Abortion Conflict.* New York: Oxford University Press.

Steinem, Gloria. 1990. "Sex, Lies, and Advertising." *Ms.,* July/August.

Turow, Joseph. 1989. *Playing Doctor: Television, Storytelling, and Medical Power.* New York: Oxford University Press.

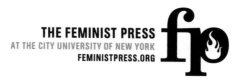